BIOMEDICAL DEVICES AND THEIR APPLICATIONS

NEW DEVELOPMENTS IN ANGIOGRAPHY RESEARCH

BIOMEDICAL DEVICES AND THEIR APPLICATIONS

Additional books in this series can be found on Nova's website under the Series tab.

Additional e-books in this series can be found on Nova's website under the e-book tab.

BIOMEDICAL DEVICES AND THEIR APPLICATIONS

NEW DEVELOPMENTS IN ANGIOGRAPHY RESEARCH

KENDRICK I. SANDERS
AND
ADDISON M. JACKSON
EDITORS

Nova Science Publishers, Inc.
New York

For permission to use material from this book please contact us:
Telephone 631-231-7269; Fax 631-231-8175
Web Site: http://www.novapublishers.com

Library of Congress Cataloging-in-Publication Data

Library of Congress Control Number: 2012935711

ISBN: 978-1-62081-492-5

Published by Nova Science Publishers, Inc. † New York

CONTENTS

PREFACE

This book provides an overview of new developments in angiography research. Topics discussed in this compilation include endovascular treatment of acute ischemic stroke; the application of CT angiography in the diagnosis of cardiovascular disease; cathether-based registration and motion compensation for 2-D/3-D fusion during electrophysiology procedures; headaches related to angiography and endovascular procedures; hybrid coronary revascularization and routine intra-operative completion angiography; and image registration techniques in Digital Subtraction Angiography (DSA).

Chapter I - Stroke is one of the most frequent causes of mortality, morbidity and disability of population in developed countries. Ischemic stroke (IS) represents 80 - 85% of all strokes in Europe and Northern America. The most often cause of IS is an acute occlusion of cerebral arteries, which can be demonstrated in more than 70% of patients in the first three to six hours after onset of symptoms. Mortality of IS patients during the first month ranges between 10% and 17% and even up to 75% in patients with malignant infarction. Finally, only about 30% of IS patients are independent after three months. These facts support the importance of IS.

Chapter II - Cardiovascular disease is the leading cause of morbidity and mortality in industrialized countries. Early detection and diagnosis are essential for improvement of treatment outcomes and patient management.

Medical imaging plays an important role in this respect, and currently computed tomography (CT) angiography has been considered the preferred imaging modality due to the emergence of multislice CT and subsequent rapid technological developments over the past decades.

The most threatening manifestations of cardiovascular disease are carotid artery stenosis, coronary artery disease, aortic dissection, aortic aneurysm, pulmonary embolism and peripheral arterial disease. This book chapter will provide an overview of the applications of CT angiography in the diagnosis of cardiovascular disease, with a focus on the diagnostic performance of CT angiography compared to invasive angiography.

Chapter III - Radio-frequency catheter ablation (RFCA) of the pulmonary veins (PVs) attached to the left atrium (LA) is usually carried out under fluoroscopy guidance. However, X-ray cannot distinguish well soft tissues, and overlay of detailed anatomical structures via 3-D CT volumes onto the fluoroscopy has shown to help visualization and navigation in Electrophysiology procedures (EP). Registration of the CT volume with the online fluoroscopy however is a challenging task for EP applications due to the lack of discernable features in fluoroscopic EP images. In addition, respiratory motion may impair the utility of static overlay of the volume with fluoroscopy for catheter navigation. In this chapter, the authors present a catheter-based method for 2-D/3-D registration and motion compensation for utilizing the 3-D data. In particular, they use the coronary sinus (CS) catheter in bi-plane fluoroscopic images and the coronary sinus in the CT volume as a location constraint to accomplish 2-D/3-D registration. After initial registration using the CS catheter, a B-spline based method for tracking the circumferential lasso catheter in monoplane fluoroscopy is implemented to track the motion at the PVs for a motion-compensated dynamic overlay. Since both the CS catheter and the lasso catheter are typically used during EP procedures, the proposed method does not require additional instruments, and achieves motion estimation right at the site of ablation. In addition, the proposed method only requires bi-plane acquisition of fluoroscopic images at the very beginning for registration purpose, and monoplane fluoroscopy is used for online monitoring and motion compensation during the EP procedures, minimizing the X-ray dose needed. The performance of the proposed tracking algorithm was evaluated on 466 monoplane frames with an average error of 0.66 ± 0.37 mms. Quantitative validation based on simulations and visual inspection on real data further demonstrates the feasibility of the proposed workflow in EP procedures.

Chapter IV - Angiography is a term which describes different techniques used to visualize the blood vessels. Computed tomography angiography, magnetic resonant angiography, and digital subtraction angiography are the vascular techniques commonly used for this purpose. These procedures are typically used to diagnose vascular abnormalities such as cerebral aneurysms, arteriovenous malformations and fistulas, cerebral vasospasm, intracranial stenosis, and vasculitis. Catheter angiography and computed tomography angiography (CTA) as well as magnetic resonance angiography (MRA) have progressively improved in the past several decades. In many situations, the noninvasive angiographic methods may be equal to catheter angiography for diagnostic accuracy. In other circumstances, conventional angiogram remains the gold standard for diagnosis of many vessel abnormalities and pathology. However, in many conditions a combination of more than one technique is reasonable and warranted for better evaluation of the vascular abnormalities. In this review, they authors will discuss some of the recent developments in angiography research and will provide updates on the new techniques in CTA, MRA, and DSA in diagnosis cerebrovascular abnormalities.

Chapter V - *Introduction*: Although many primary headaches are attributed to structural and functional changes of intracranial vessels, studies on pain from direct stimulation of the arterial or venous walls are scarce. Intracranial endovascular procedures can be viewed as models to study that type of pain. On the other hand, the occurrence of headaches during and after endovascular procedures can be a red flag for an intracranial complication or simply a consequence of vessel manipulation.

Purpose: In this chapter the authors review the data about headaches related to angiography and endovascular procedures and try to correlate their mechanisms and localization. They also attempt to characterize clinically these headaches, in order to identify relevant clinical alarm signs for evaluation of headaches related to endovascular procedures.

Methods: A review of publications in English, French or Portuguese language with the key words vascular headache, headache, migraine, angiography, embolization, endovascular interventions was sought. Primary headaches were excluded.

Results: Headache occurs frequently (19 to 65%) during angiography and endovascular procedures, always in consequence of a specific manoeuvre and it is sharp, intense, brief without accompanying symptoms. It projects to the scalp area in the distribution of the nocipetive innervation of the involved artery. Headache frequently (33 to 47%) appears in the 24 hours after angiography and it is usually self-limited, mild and uncharacteristic. Angiography and endovascular procedures do not increase the likelihood of future recurrent headaches.

Chapter VI - Hybrid coronary revascularization combines coronary artery bypass grafting (CABG) surgery with percutaneous coronary intervention (PCI) for coronary artery disease. Surgical grafting is reserved for revascularization of the left anterior descending (LAD) artery, usually performed with the left internal mammary artery (LIMA) through either a limited thoracotomy or an endoscopic approach, while PCI with stenting is reserved for revascularization of non-LAD lesions. This combines the benefits of each technique—namely, the superiority of the LIMA to LAD graft and the improved patency rate of stent placement in non-LAD vessels. For non-LAD vessels, the higher one-year failure rate for saphenous vein grafts (SVG, averages 20%) compared to drug-eluting stents (DES, average 9%) supports this hybrid approach.

The hybrid procedure can be performed as a staged procedure—with PCI followed by CABG or CABG followed by PCI. However, hybrid coronary revascularization is increasingly performed as a combined ("one stop") procedure in a dedicated suite—the "hybrid operating room". The hybrid room has the capability of serving both as a complete surgical operating room and as a catheterization laboratory.

The hybrid operating room also allows for routine completion angiography following CABG surgery. This facilitates early identification of graft failure thereby providing the opportunity to correct technical errors within the same surgical period and thus may improve graft patency rate, especially of SVG to non-LAD vessels. This chapter reviews the advantages of and the logistics required for performing hybrid procedures and completion angiography—a new horizon for coronary surgery.

Chapter VII - Image registration is one of the most important image processing operations in Digital Subtraction Angiography (DSA). In this application, it is necessary to register multiple images of the same sequence in order to reduce patient motion artifacts. The registered images are then subtracted in order to evaluate the progress of a disease and/or a treatment procedure. In this chapter, a follow-up of some recent automatic registration techniques for digital X-ray angiography images is presented. A first method is based on a 3-D space-time motion evaluation and on an edge-detection approach leading to the selection of a set of control points from which pixels having their values changed due to motion are separated from those due to contrast flow, by means of detecting the peak iodine opacification. A second technique is based on local similarity detection by means of template matching according to the combined invariants-based similarity measure. The main characteristic of the third approach is that it combines the two previous ones to establish correspondences between the potentially matched movement points detected from the two images. The results clearly indicate that the third registration algorithm is much better able to recover patient motion than the other ones and would therefore be the method of choice for automatic registration of angiographic images.

In: New Developments in Angiography Research
Editors: K. I. Sanders and A. M. Jackson

ISBN: 978-1-62081-492-5

Chapter I

Endovascular Treatment of Acute Ischemic Stroke

T. Jonszta[1], M. Kuliha[2], M. Roubec[2], R. Herzig[3], D. Šaňák[3], V. Procházka[1] and D. Školoudík[2,3,*]

[1]Comprehensive Stroke Center, Department of Radiology, University Hospital Ostrava, Ostrava, Czech Republic
[2]Comprehensive Stroke Center, Department of Neurology, University Hospital Ostrava, Ostrava, Czech Republic
[3]Comprehensive Stroke Center, Department of Neurology, Faculty of Medicine and Dentistry, Palacký University and University Hospital, Olomouc, Czech Republic

Introduction

Stroke is one of the most frequent causes of mortality, morbidity and disability of population in developed countries. [1,2] Ischemic stroke (IS) represents 80 - 85% of all strokes in Europe and Northern America. The most often cause of IS is an acute occlusion of cerebral arteries, which can be demonstrated in more than 70% of patients in the first three to six hours after onset of symptoms. [3] Mortality of IS patients during the first month ranges between 10% and 17% and even up to 75% in patients with malignant infarction. [4] Finally, only about 30% of IS patients are independent after three months. [2] These facts support the importance of IS.

The location of cerebral artery occlusion and time to recanalization are known independent prognostic factors of IS. Early recanalization within six hours after onset of symptoms is associated with a significantly higher chance of independency after 90 days with a significant reduction of mortality [5].

* Address for correspondence: Assoc. Prof. David Školoudík, MD, PhD, FESO. Comperhensive Stroke Center. Department of Neurology, University Hospital Ostrava, CZ-708 52 Ostrava-Poruba , Czech Republic.

Table 1. Thrombectomy devices for acute stroke in use [14]

Device Class	Company Name	FDA Indication	In Clinical Use?
Aspiration/Suction			
Amplatz Thrombectomy	Ev3 Medical	Mechanical dissolution of thrombus within dialysis fistulae	No longer marketed
AngioJet	Possis	Breaking apart or removing of thrombus in peripheral veins or arterio-venous access conduits	Yes
NeuroJet	Possis	N/A	No longer marketed
Oasis Thrombectomy	Boston Scientific	Removing thrombus from hemodialysis access grafts	No longer marketed
Penumbra	Penumbra, Inc	Revascularization of patients with acute ischemic stroke	Yes
Vasco +35	Balt Extrusion	N/A	Not in US
Clot Retriever			
Attractor-18	Boston Scientific	N/A	No longer marketed
Catch	Balt Extrusion	N/A	Not in US
In-Time	Boston Scientific	Retrieval of intravascular foreign objects in peripheral vascular, neurovasculature and cardiovasculature	No longer marketed
MERCI	Concentric Medical	Restore blood flow in the neurovasculature	Yes
Phenox	Phenox GmbH	N/A	Not in US
TriSpan	Boston Scientific	N/A	No longer marketed
Ultrasonography			
EKOS	EKOS Corporation	Infusion of fluids into peripheral vasculature	Yes
OmniWave	OmniSonics	Removal of thrombus and infusion of fluids into peripheral vasculature	No longer marketed
Snare			
Alligator	Chestnut Medici Technologies, Inc.	Peripheral and neurovasculature foreign body removal	Yes
Amplatz Gooseneck	Ev3 Medical	Retrieval and manipulation of atraumatic foreign bodls in coronary and peripheral cardiovascular system and the extra-cranial neurovascular anatomy	Yes
Device Class	Company Name	FDA Indication	In Clinical Use?
EnSnare Device	Merit Medici Systems, Inc.	Retrieval and manipulation of foreign objects in the cardiovascular system or hollow viscous	Yes
Neuronet	Boston Scientific	N/A	No longer marketed
Soutenir	Solution	N/A	Not in US
Laser			
EPAR	Endovasix Inc.	N/A	No longer marketed
LaTIS	Spectranetics	Removal of thrombus from vascular grafts	No longer marketed

EPAR - Endovascular Photoacoustic Recanalization, FDA—Food and Drug Administration, NA—not applicable, US—United States.

In the last decade, the number of methods used for acceleration of artery recanalization strongly increased. In addition to pharmacological methods, especially intravenous (IVT) and intra-arterial thrombolysis (IAT) [6-8], mechanical (neuro-interventional) methods (i.e., Merci Retrieval System®, Penumbra System®, Solitaire® stent, Trevo Pro®, Catch device®, Phenox Clot Retriever®, BONNET Intracranial Flow Restoration Device®, pRESET Thrombectomy Retriever®, direct stent placement, EkoSonicTM Endovascular System, In-Time™ Retrieval Device, Amplatz Goose-Neck MicroSnare®, Attracter-18™, Neuronet™ Guidant device, LaTIS laser device®, Possis Angiojet system®) were tested and introduced into clinical practice similarly as in the treatment of heart ischemic syndromes—Table 1 [9-14].

Data from the meta-analysis of 53 clinical trials (including 2,066 patients) suggests that early recanalization is present only in 24.1% patients without specific treatment (spontaneous recanalization), 46.2% patients treated with IVT, 63.2% patients treated with IAT, 67.5% of patients treated with combined IVT - IAT and in up to 83.6% patients treated with mechanical methods [5]. Endovascular therapy as a new early recanalization option for patients with acute IS is currently intensely investigated. Nevertheless, the use of these methods only in specialized centers represents the main limitation.

Several thrombectomy devices will be introduced with results of studies and a list of ongoing trials.

THROMBECTOMY DEVICES

Merci Retriever (Concentric Medical, Mountain View, CA, US)

The Merci Retrieval System® is a minimally invasive catheter-based system designed to retrieve and remove clots in patients experiencing acute IS. It was one of the first thrombectomy systems used in acute stroke patients. The Merci Retrieval System® consists of three parts: Merci retriever, Merci microcatheter and Merci balloon guide catheter—Figure 1.

The Merci Retrievers® are constructed from nitinol (nickel titanium) memory-wire and are corkscrew-shaped. This design is considered to be best suited for blood clot removal from large vessels within the neurovasculature. The Merci Retriever® is delivered through the dedicated Merci® MC18L microcatheter to the lesion location in its linear formation. Once deployed, the retriever returns to its coiled shape to ensnare and retrieve the clot. The Merci Retrievers are compatible with the Merci® Balloon Guide Catheter. This catheter comes in two sizes—namely 8 and 9F. The catheter has compliant silicone balloon mounted at its end. The balloon soft and atraumatic design provides temporary flow arrest in thrombectomy procedures when inflated. This should help to prevent distal embolization. One lumen is used to inflate and deflate the balloon, while the second lumen allows continuous access to the neuro vasculature.

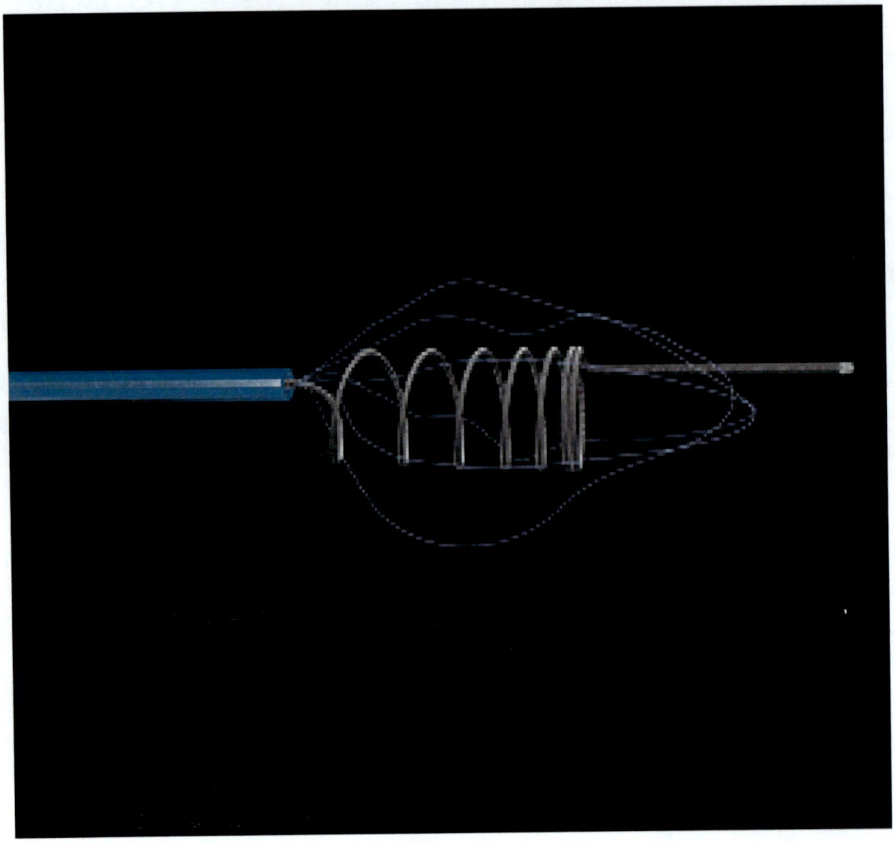

Figure 1. Merci V Retriever® (Concentric Medical, Mountain View, CA, US).

There are currently ten Merci Retrievers® available to match different vessel sizes. The newest generation of Retrievers®, the V Series, incorporates features of the two earlier generations to create a best-in-class thrombectomy device. The V Series is designed such that the proximal loops stretch to engage the clot, while the two distal loops remain intact to capture the clot.

Merci Retrievers® are also indicated for use in the retrieval of foreign bodies misplaced during interventional radiological procedures in the neuro, peripheral and coronary vasculature.

The Merci Retriever® was first cleared for human use in 2004, by the Food and Drug Administration (FDA). Since 2004, the Merci Retriever® has been used in more than 14,000 patients throughout the world including the United States, Europe, Australia, Singapore and Canada, and since May 2010, also in Japan.

Published Studies

Successive generations of the MERCI device have been reported in three prospective, single-arm, nonrandomized, multicenter feasibility and safety studies. In the MERCI-I trial, 28 patients were treated with this technique with 64% successful recanalizations. In the following prospective, nonrandomized, multicenter MERCI II trial, the safety and efficacy of a novel embolectomy device (Merci Retriever) to open occluded intracranial large vessels within eight hours of the onset of stroke symptoms were tested. All patients were ineligible for intravenous recombinant tissue plasminogen activator (rt-PA). Recanalization was achieved in 46% of patients on intention to treat analysis. This rate was significantly higher than 18% in historical controls of ($P < 0.0001$). Clinically significant procedural complications occurred in 7.1% patients. Symptomatic intracranial hemorrhages (SICH) were observed in 7.8% patients. Good neurological outcomes (defined as a modified Rankin scale [mRS] 0-2) were observed in 46% patients versus 10% in historical controls (relative risk 4.4, $P < 0.0001$) and mortality was in 32% patients versus 54% in historical controls (relative risk 0.59, $P < 0.01$) [15].

The results were confirmed in the Multi MERCI international, multicenter, prospective, single-arm trial. One hundred and sixty-four patients with large vessel IS who had received IV rt-PA but did not recanalize or who were ineligible for IV rt-PA and were treated within eight hours of symptom onset were included in the study. Treatment with the Retriever alone resulted in successful recanalization in 57.3% treatable vessels and in 69.5% after adjunctive therapy (IA rt-PA, mechanical). SICH occurred in 9.0%. Clinically significant procedural complications occurred in 5.5% patients [16]. There was no definite association between time to treatment or reperfusion and outcomes in the unadjusted analysis. After adjustment for age, baseline NIHSS, and glucose, there was a strong trend toward fewer independent outcomes with later reperfusion times [17].

Final recanalization status was the strongest predictor of clinical outcomes in patients undergoing thrombectomy in presented studies. The ability to remove the clot was negatively influenced by systolic blood pressure [18].

Post hoc analysis with patients in the MERCI (68 patients) and Multi MERCI (81 patients) trials, who would have been eligible for PROACT II, showed a trend toward better clinical outcomes compared to the PROACT II control arm. In both unadjusted and adjusted analyses, mortality rates did not significantly differ between embolectomy patients and PROACT II control patients [19]. No statistically significant differences were found between patients with occlusion of M2-segment of middle cerebral artery (MCA) and M1-segment of MCA for symptomatic hemorrhage, clinically significant procedural adverse events, favorable 90-day outcome, or 90-day mortality. In multivariate analysis, final revascularization was the strongest independent predictor of good outcome at 90 days [20].

Further analysis showed that mechanical thrombectomy of acute intracranial internal carotid artery (ICA) occlusion using the Merci Retriever device, alone or in combination with adjunctive endovascular therapy, has a high rate of successful vessel recanalization (39%). Subjects with successful ICA recanalization by this method have improved post-stroke clinical outcome and survival compared with subjects in whom the ICA is not successfully recanalized [21]. Patients with vertebrobasilar occlusion in the MERCI and Multi-MERCI trials achieved recanalization in 78% cases, mortality was 44% and good outcomes were seen in 41%. Outcomes in these patients compared favorably with natural history reports. Patients with recanalization tended to have better outcomes than those without [22].

Penumbra System® (Penumbra Inc., Alameda, CA, US)

Penumbra Inc.'s IS device platform, the Penumbra System® (Figure 2), is designed to revascularize or open up a blood vessel that is blocked by a blood clot. The Penumbra System® is FDA cleared and CE–marked. The system is based on a continuous aspiration thrombectomy platform. It includes reperfusion microcatheter that is connected to an aspiration pump through aspiration tubing, generating a suction force of -700 mm Hg. A teardrop-shaped separator is advanced and retracted within the lumen of the reperfusion catheter to debulk the clot for ease of aspiration. As a nonpharmacologic tool, it has the potential of reopening a vessel without the use of adjunctive thrombolytics, thus offering dual options for recanalization via a single access platform. In addition, the system is designed to minimize the need to blindly penetrate into the occluded vascular segment because it operates from the proximal end of the clot. Due to the flexibility and variety of available sizes (0.26 – 0.54 inch) of the reperfusion microcatheters, even smaller distal branches such as M2 and A2 can be successfully accessed for recanalization.

Published Studies

The phase 1 trial showed a 100% revascularization rate to TIMI 2 or 3 in 20 patients (21 vessels). The pivotal phase 2 trial, completed in September 2007, showed a TIMI 2 or 3 recanalization rate of 81.6% with a low periprocedural serious adverse event score of 3.4% in 125 patients treated with this device; none were device-related. SICH occurred in 11.2% of the patients, and all-cause mortality was 32.8%. Good neurologic outcome as (defined as a > 4 points improvement on the NIHSS score at discharge) was observed in 57.8% of the patients, whereas good functional outcome as defined by a 90-day mRS score of zero to two was reported in 25% of patients. Patients who were successfully recanalized by the Penumbra System® had generally better outcomes than those who were not [23,24].

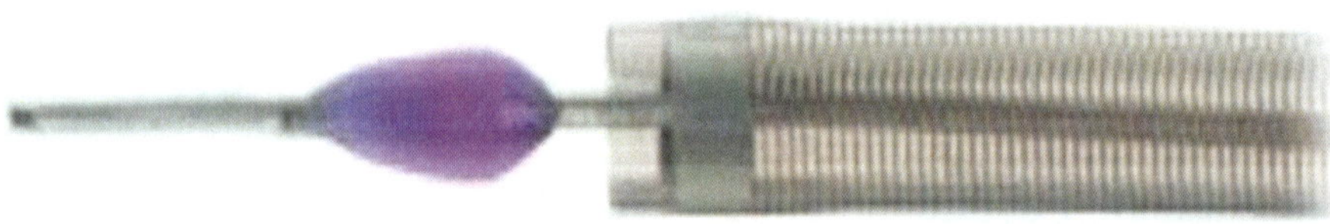

Figure 2. Penumbra System® (Penumbra Inc., Alameda, CA, US).

First single-center experiences as well as preliminary data from the first post-market multicenter study seemed to confirm these findings. In a retrospective case review study performed in 139 patients treated by the Penumbra System® at seven centers in the United States and Europe, the device was found to successfully recanalize the target vessel in 84% of cases, with similar outcome and intracranial hemorrhage rates as those in the pivotal trial. In fact, 40% of the patients had achieved a mRS score of ≤ 2 at 90 days, which is a significantly higher rate than that reported earlier [25]. Thus, it appears that the favorable safety and effectiveness profile of the Penumbra System® observed in the pivotal trial can be extended to the real-world setting.

Solitaire™ Stent (Ev3, Irvine, CA, US)

Solitaire™ AB (FR) Neurovascular Remodeling Device is the only fully deployable and completely retrievable self-expanding stent designed for bridging the neck of aneurysms. It can be fully retrieved, even when fully deployed, repositioned and redeployed again—Figures 3 a,b.

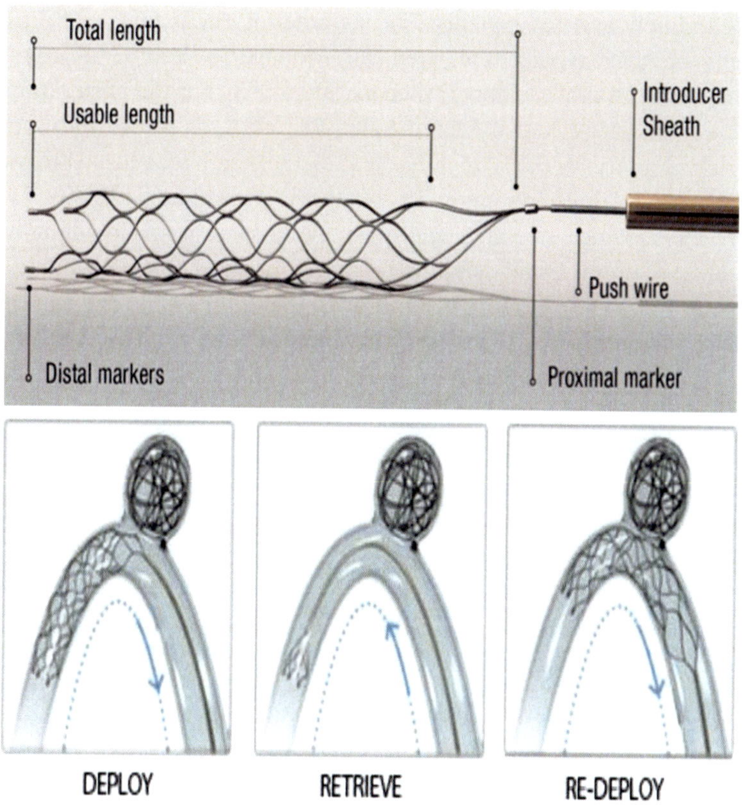

Figure 3 a,b. Solitaire™ AB (FR) Neurovascular Remodeling Device (Ev3, Irvine, CA, US).

Solitaire™ AB (FR) stent is deployed through a standard 0.021" or 0.027" micro catheter on a 0.016" pushwire, which means that Solitaire™ AB (FR) delivers just like an intracranial coil. It allows multiple retrievals, even after full deployment for adjustment and superior placement. It can be introduced easily even into very tortuous vessels. Its open slit, closed-cell design gives Solitaire AB an optimal radial force with good kink resistance. It can be deployed by electrolytic detachment. It is available in two diameters of 4 or 6 mm and lengths 26, 31 and 41 mm.

As per the manufacturer's recommendation, this stent is designed for the treatment of intracranial neurovascular disease. At first, it was intended for wide neck aneurysm treatment only. At present, it is also renowned for its excellent results in intracranial vessel recanalization in stroke patients.

The unique Solitaire™ stent design features allow dual functionality: firstly, it acts as a temporary intracranial bypass providing immediate flow restoration through the thrombus after the temporary stent deployment. Secondly, it acts as a clot retriever, trapping thrombus into its cells allowing the clot removal. It received CE Mark approval as a flow restoration device.

Procedure

All procedures are performed via a femoral artery approach under sedation or in general anesthesia in extremely agitated patients. For the anterior circulation, an 8 Fr or 9 Fr Merci balloon guiding catheter (Concentric Medical, Mountain View, CA, US) is introduced through a femoral sheath into the appropriate carotid artery. For the posterior circulation, a 6 Fr Envoy guiding catheter (Cordis, Miami Lake, FL, USA) is placed into the dominant, or navigable, vertebral artery. A 0.021 inch internal diameter microcatheter Prowler Select Plus (Cordis) or Vasco 21 (Balt, Montmorency, France) is navigated distally to the point of occlusion over a 0.014 inch steerable microwire. A microcatheter angiographic run is then carried out in order to confirm and define the vasculature distal to the thrombus.

The Solitaire™ AB (FR) is introduced through the 0,021" microcatheter, and the device is deployed across the occluding thrombus. The microcatheter is then partially withdrawn, so that the distal marker is positioned at the exact level of the proximal marker of the stent. After the Solitaire™ AB (FR) deployment, an angiographic control is performed in order to evaluate the correct placement and expansion of the stent and to find out if there already is flow restoration past the occlusion site. After the angiographic run, the Solitaire™ AB (FR) is maintained in place for a few (three to seven) minutes to allow device expansion. After this time, the stent is slightly resheathed and then both the deployed Solitaire™ AB and the delivery microcatheter are gently pulled back together and recovered through the guiding catheter. Immediately after the retrieval, it is necessary to aspirate the content of the guiding catheter in order to remove any clot debris eventually present in the lumen of the guiding catheter. In case of unsuccessful thrombus removal, another attempt is usually indicated. After thorough cleaning of the stent, it can be reintroduced into occlusion site. If necessary, up to five passes are performed using the device. The integrity of the stent must be consistently checked after every pass. In case of repeated unsuccessful thrombus retrieval, suboptimal angiographic result in atherosclerotic lesions or inability to recapture the stent, a bail-out option of repositioning the stent is available following with permanent deploying it by electrolytic detachment, similar to coil. However, its radial force is not very high, and very often different types of stents need to be used to finish the procedure.

Mechanical thrombectomy also has its specific potential drawbacks. It usually takes a longer time compared to direct stenting. There is also increased risk of intimal injury to the vessel wall while withdrawing an unfolded stent to perform thrombectomy. It luckily proved to be of little concern in the clinical setting. However, microscopic studies have proved some minor intimal injuries in animal studies. Vasospasms and subarachnoidal hemorrhage have been described in clinical studies after thrombectomy with the Solitaire device.

Published Studies

Current reports with Solitaire device come from different European centers since the device is not currently approved in the United States. Castano et al. [26] reported their experience in the treatment of 20 patients with acute IS and large vessel occlusion in the anterior circulation. Recanalization grade TICI 2b/3 was achieved in 90% of treated vessels, and no procedural complications were reported. SICH occurred in 10% of patients, and 45% of them achieved a mRS ≤ 2 at three months. The device used in this study was the Solitaire AB stent, initially designed as an aneurysm neck bridging stent. The device was deployed for one or two min before retrieving it to perform embolectomy. Recanalization required in average 1.4 passes. The successful off-label use of this stent prompted the creation of the Solitaire™ FR device with minimal modifications from the AB version and specifically designed for treatment of acute IS.

Machi et al. [27] achieved successful recanalization in 50 out of the 56 patients (89%) treated with the Solitaire™ FR device. Procedure-related complications occurred in 9% of patients, and 46% of them achieved a mRS $\leq$ 2 at discharge. The mean number of passes required per procedure was two (1–5 range). The device was positioned across the area of occlusion for three to seven min and then gently recovered into the guide catheter. Vasospasm during retrieval of the fully deployed stent was a common phenomenon; two patients had asymptomatic subarachnoidal hemorrhage and one patient, SICH.

Similarly, Roth et al. [28] treated 22 patients with acute IS and achieved TICI flow 2a/b or 3 in 91% of patients. Two SICH occurred, and 50% of patients achieved a mRS ≤ 2 at 90 days. Vasospasm after thrombectomy was noticed in three patients, and no device-related complications were reported.

Seifert et al. [29] reported experience with a Solitaire™ device in conjunction with IVT or IAT in four patients, achieving TIMI grade 2 to 3 recanalization in all patients and clinical improvement (median mRS, one at 30 days) in 50%. There was one death, and the other patient was lost to follow-up.

Investigators of the REscue, COmbined, and Stand-alone Thrombectomy (RECOST) study achieved TICI 3 flow in 84% of patients with acute IS treated with the Solitaire™ FR/AB device. [30] The aim of this study was to evaluate and appraise the timing, safety and efficacy of an integrated stroke management protocol. At three months, 54% of patients achieved a mRS ≤ 2 and 2% had SICH. The device was deployed for two to seven min in the target occlusion before thrombectomy.

Case Report 1

A 74-year-old male was admitted to the hospital (stroke center) with left-sided hemiparesis, left-side facial palsy, dysarthria, eye deviation and neglect syndrome (NIHSS 14 points). Computed tomography angiography (CTA) finding confirmed T-occlusion of the distal ICA, anterior cerebral artery (ACA) and middle cerebral artery (MCA) on the right side. Atrial fibrillation treated with Aspirin® 100 mg daily, arterial hypertension and hypercholesterolemia were in medical history. Patient was treated with IVT (90 mg of rt-PA) 140 minutes after stroke onset. Patient's clinical status did not improve during IVT; therefore, he was transferred to angiography for mechanical recanalization. Persistent T-occlusion of the ICA was detected (Figure 4a). Successful thrombectomy with Solitaire™ device was performed, and the vessels were recanalized completely five hours after onset of symptoms (Figures 4 b-d). At discharge, patient presented with residual mild left-sided hemiparesis (mRS 2); small ischemic area in the right basal ganglia was shown by computer tomography (CT).

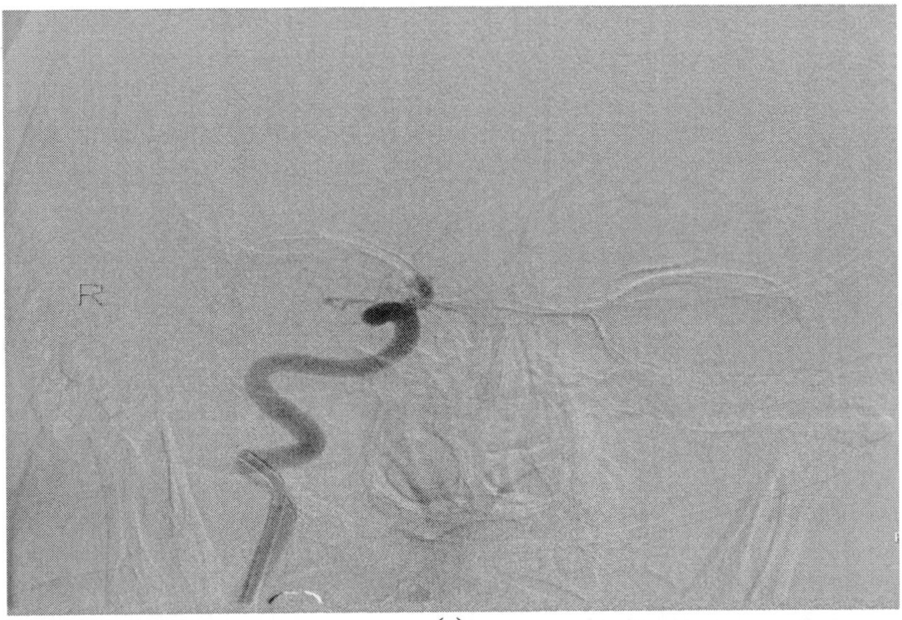

(a)

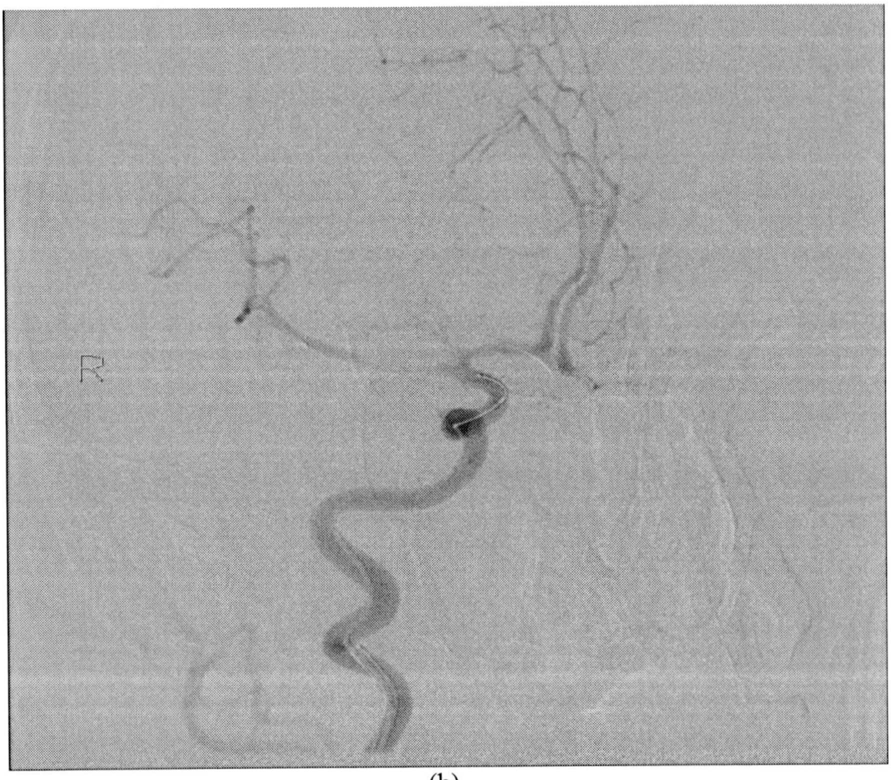

(b)

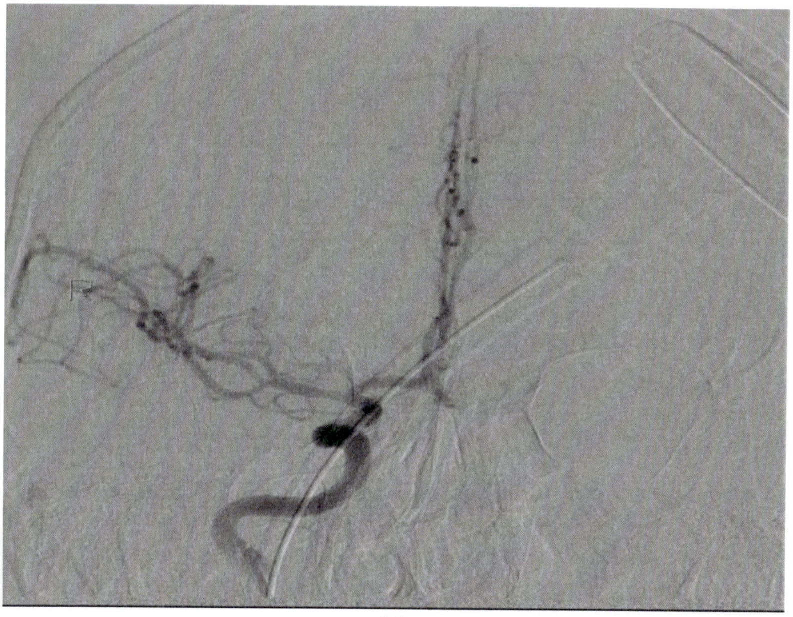

(c)

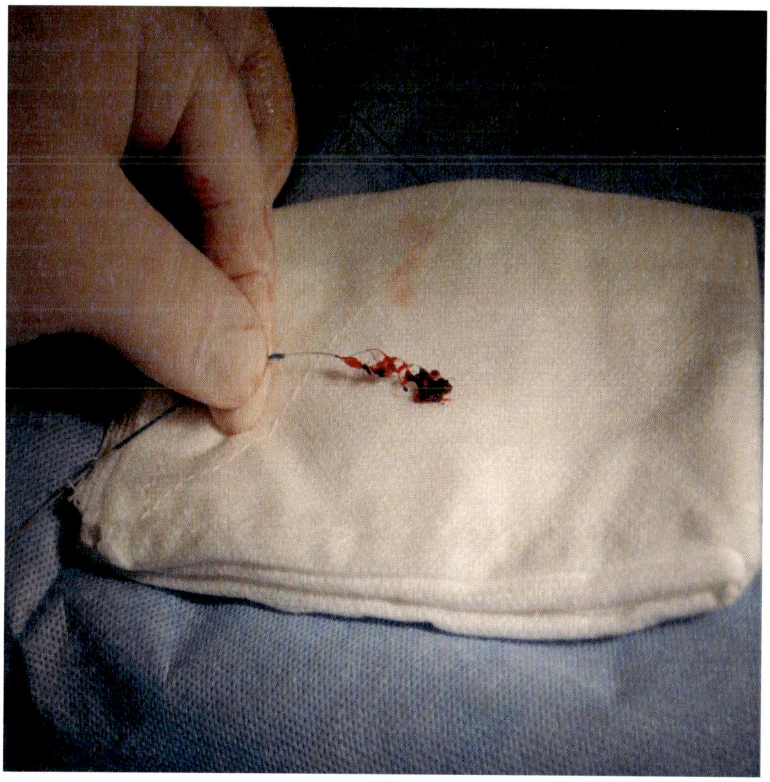

(d)

Figures 4 a-d. Recanalization of middle cerebral artery using Solitaire™ stent: Distal occlusion of internal carotid artery (4a). Solitaire stent deployed in the middle cerebral artery - flow restoration also called temporary bypass (4b). Middle cerebral artery recanalization after successful thrombectomy (4c). Solitaire stent immediately after extraction with thrombi in stent struts (4d).

Trevo Pro® (Concentric Medical, Mountain View, CA, US)

The Trevo System® is a non-deployable, sized 4 x 20mm stent-like device currently used in Europe and Canada. Its body is very soft and allows easy navigation through tortuous vessels, and its distal closed-end is intended to prevent vessel perforation—Figures 5 a,b. The device can be used in vessels ranging from 1.5 to 3.5 mm in diameter. The orientation of the stent struts has the thinner portion of the struts facing the vessel lumen in order to optimize thrombus incorporation, opposite to the design of stents used to treat intracranial aneurysms or intracranial atherosclerosis.

The Trevo System® is being introduced into the occluded vessel via a 0.021" inner diameter large microcatheter. The deployment and clot extraction should be performed in a similar manner to that of Solitaire™ stent. The system is currently under investigation in pivotal study named Trevo 2 Clinical Trial. [31]

Mendonça et al. published results of a prospective study with 13 acute stroke patients (eight patients with MCA and five patients with ICA occlusion) treated by Trevo system®. Revascularization was achieved in 77% patients without periprocedural complications. Four patients (30%) died during the 90-day follow-up period and four patients (30%) achieved functional independence [32].

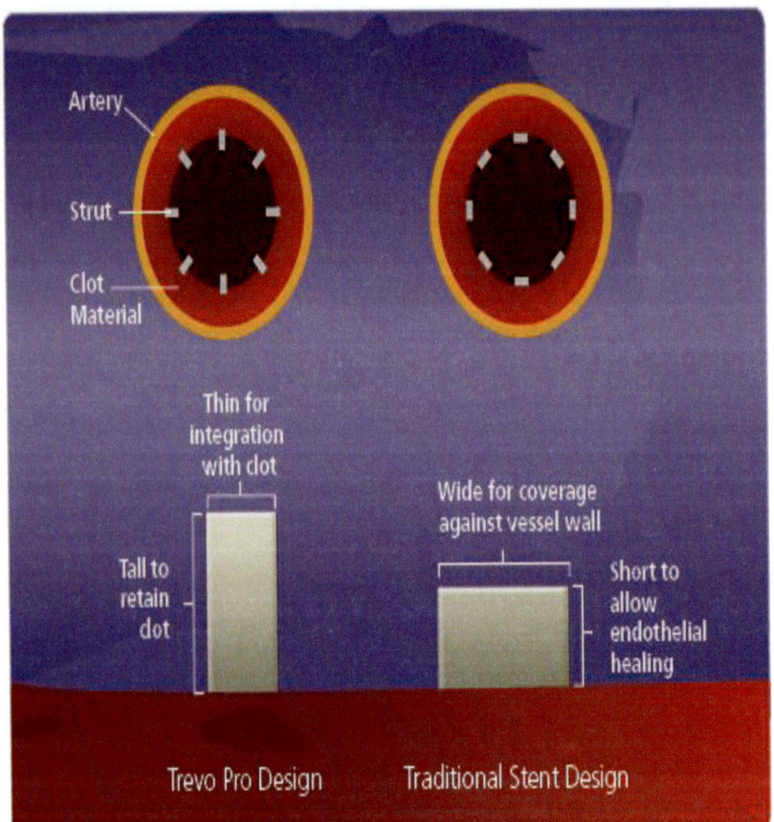

(a)

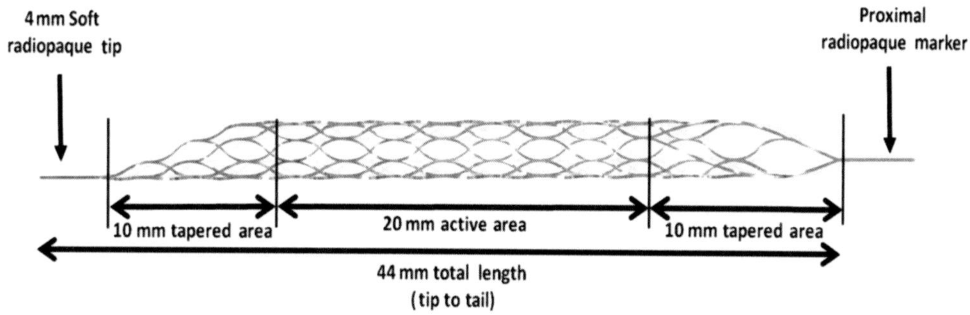

(b)

Figure 5 a,b. Trevo Pro® (Concentric Medical, Mountain View, CA, US).

2.5. Catch Device® (Balt Extrusion, Montmorency, France)

The Catch Device® owes its design to Leo stent and is made of Nitinol. In fact, it looks like tiny wire basket intended for thrombus retrieval—Figure 6. Its external diameter is 4 millimeters, and the device is intended for use in vessels of diameter up to 5 millimeters. This device must be introduced exclusively by microcatheter Vasco+21, which has internal diameter of 0.0236". The microcatheter must be positioned at least 2 cm downstream behind the thrombus. Then the basket is opened, and the whole system can be withdrawn through 6F guiding catheter. However, the Catch basket cannot be resheathed into the Vasco microcatheter. Mourand et al. published results of retrospective study with 40 consecutive acute IS patients. Recanalization (TIMI grade 2 – 3) was achieved in 65% cases. SICH occurred in 18% cases. Periprocedural complications occurred in 15% patients without clinical consequences: four clot fragmentations and two vasospasms. Good functional outcome (mRS ≤ 2) after 90 days was achieved in 39% patients. Good functional outcome at 90 days was more frequent (56.5 vs. 7.7%), and mortality rate was lower (30.0 vs. 61.5%) in patients with successful recanalization in comparison with patients with unsuccessful recanalization [33].

Phenox Clot Retriever® (Phenox GmbH, Bochum, Germany)

This Germany-based company offers a whole range of unique-design mechanical thrombectomy systems.

Phenox clot retriever - pCR® is a device with a brush-like structure—Figure 7. The fibre structure made from nylon (polyamide) filaments increases in diameter from proximal to distal end. The fibres have also X-ray markers at the both distal and proximal ends. The fibre work, which has large surface area for efficient thrombus removal, is connected to a three-meter-long guiding wire, which is introduced into the body through a micro-catheter. This system is 22 millimetres long and is available in three different diameters intended to treat vessels ranging in diameter from 1 to above 3 millimeters. The pCR is introduced through microcatheter. Upon deployment behind the occluding thrombus, the filaments unfold, and the thrombus is captured in the fibre network. The system is then gradually withdrawn into the guiding catheter under constant aspiration and removed.

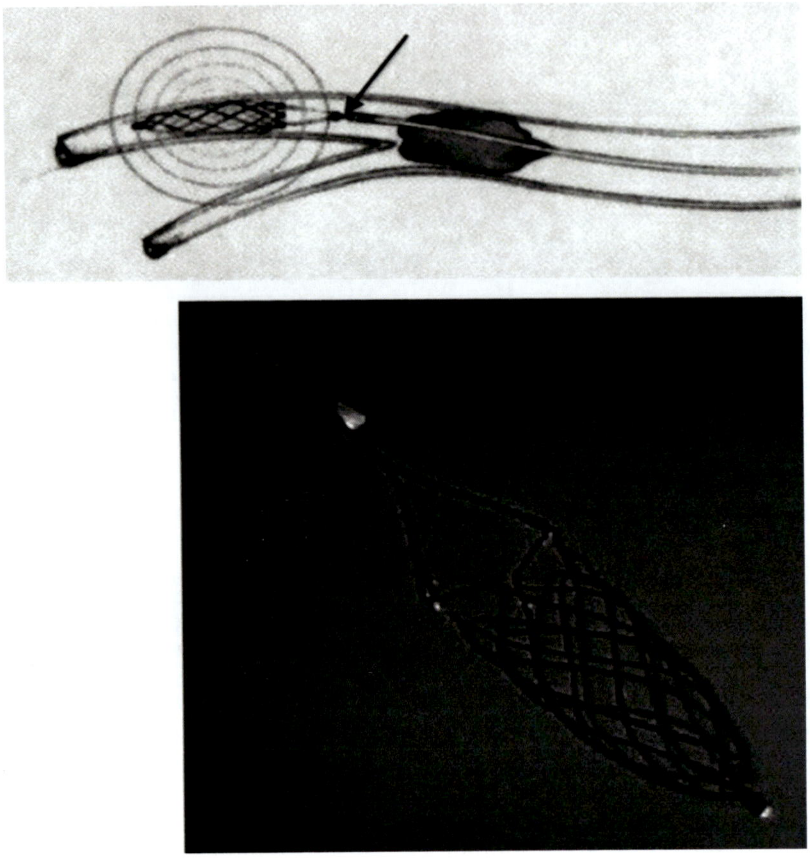

Figure 6. Catch device® (Balt Extrusion, Montmorency, France).

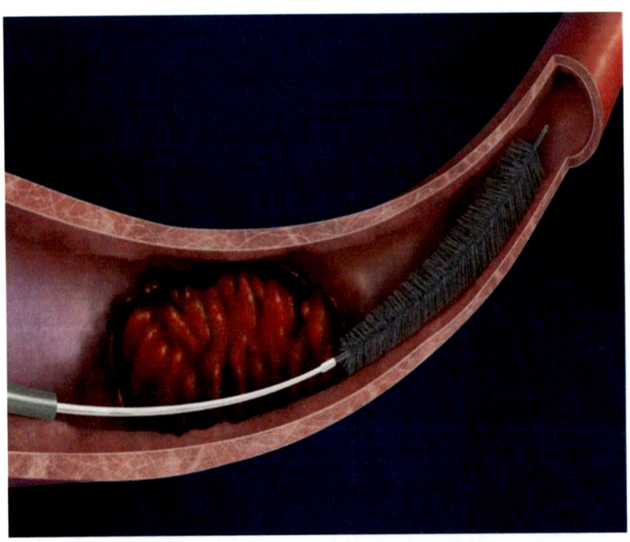

Figure 7. Phenox clot retriever - pCR® (Phenox GmbH, Bochum, Germany).

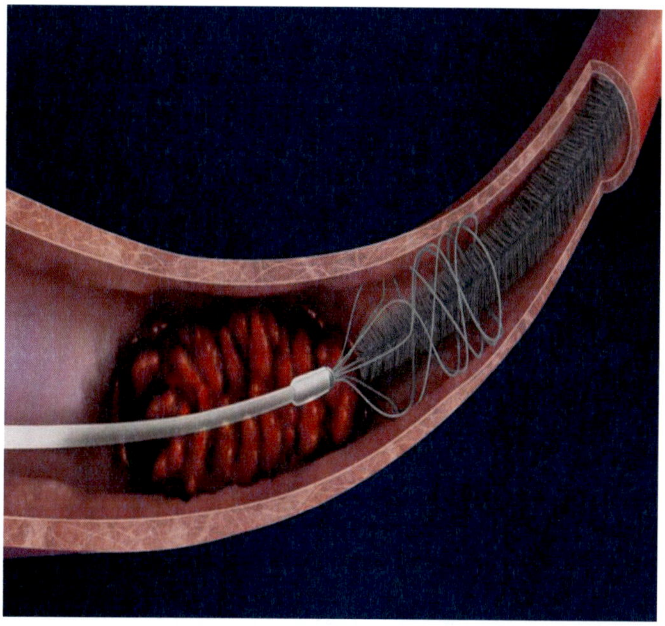

Figure 8. CRC phenox Clot Retriever CAGE® (Phenox GmbH, Bochum, Germany).

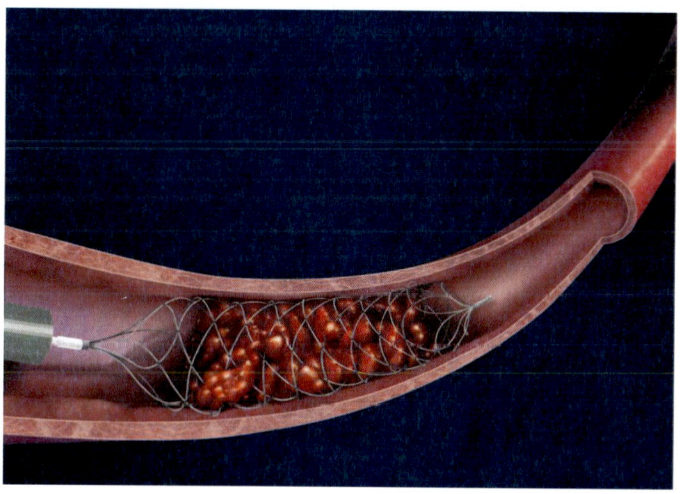

Figure 9. BONNET Intracranial Flow Restoration Device® (Phenox GmbH, Bochum, Germany).

CRC phenox Clot Retriever CAGE®, like the pCR, is made from a fibre work of polyamide filaments. In contrast to the pCR, the CRC possesses an additional Nitinol (nickel, titanium) thread cage at the proximal end of its fibre brush—Figure 8. This nitinol cage gives a higher radial range, which is an advantage against older and/or firmer thrombi. This system is available in two different sizes intended to treat vessels with diameter ranging from 2 to above 3 millimetres. Otherwise, the design of the polyamide fibres, central wire, insertion wire and system markers is identical to the pCR system. The system insertion, deployment and final thrombus removal is also performed in the same way.

Both the pCR and the CRC systems are intended for single extraction only, which means that they must be exchanged for different devices in case of first attempt extraction failure.

Bonnet Intracranial Flow Restoration Device® (Phenox GmbH, Bochum, Germany)

The BONNET Intracranial Flow Restoration Device® consists of a self-expanding nitinol braiding with polyamide filaments passing through the interior—Figure 9. These enlarge the surface area and enable better fixation of the thrombus mass. The instrument is firmly connected with an insertion wire, and carries X-ray visible markers at its proximal and distal ends. The size of this device is 5 x 35 mm.

The BONNET® has high flexibility and is easy to advance through tortuous vessels. It is also a repeatedly re-usable device. The system is advanced through microcatheter and should preferably be deployed distally of the thrombus. However, it can also be released after withdrawal of the micro-catheter partially or completely into the thrombus. The micro-catheter does not have to be completely removed. The flow restoration is achieved through simultaneous withdrawal of the BONNET® and the micro-catheter through the guiding catheter. The system can either be put distally of the thrombus or can be released into the thrombus. Re-use in the same patient is possible, for example in another vessel blockage.

The BONNET short Intracranial Flow Restoration Device® is a new variant of the trusted BONNET®. In addition to its new size, the system displays a new shape and a higher level of relative radial force. The BONNET short® consists of a self-expanding nitinol braiding with polyamide filaments passing through the interior—Figure 10. The system is firmly connected with an insertion wire in an eccentric attachment and carries X-ray visible markers at its proximal and distal ends. It enables a fast and safe intracranial vessel flow restoration also in curved vessel areas. Re-use in the same patient is possible, for example in another vessel blockage. Its size is 5 x 23 mm, and it is suitable for vessels larger than 2 mm. The technique of its deployment and withdrawal is the same as in BONNET system®.

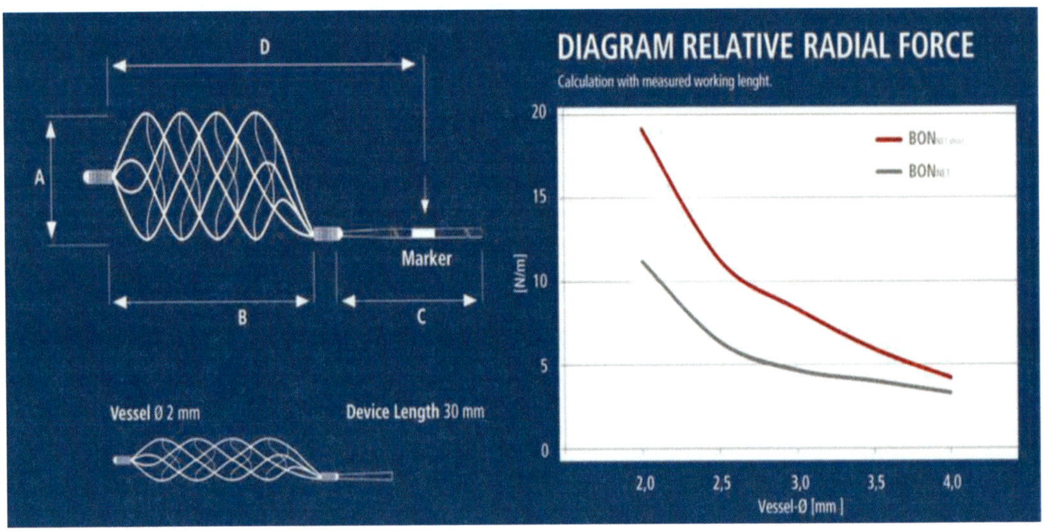

Figure 10. BONNET short Intracranial Flow Restoration Device® (Phenox GmbH, Bochum, Germany).

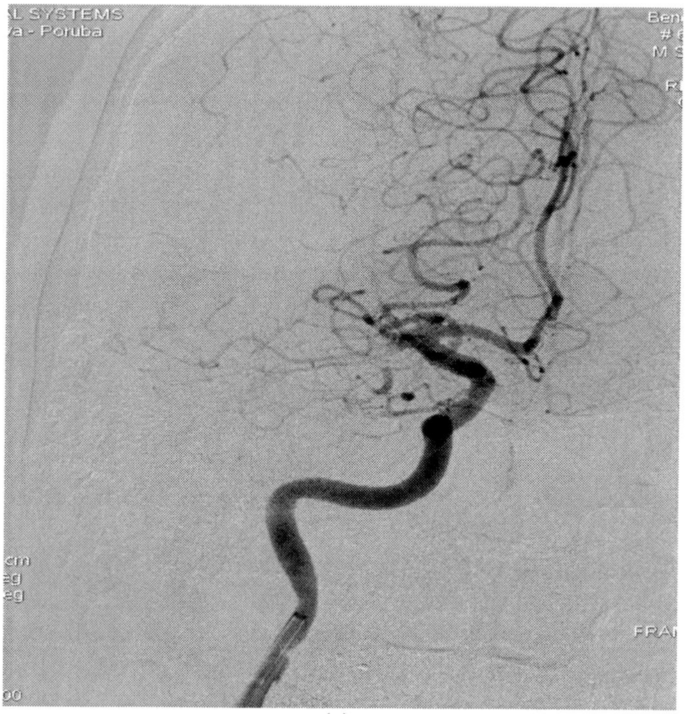

(a)

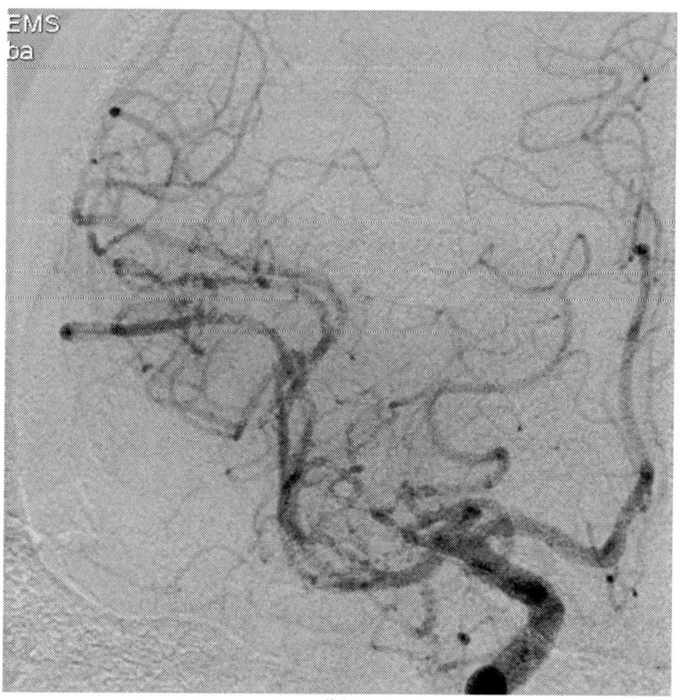

(b)

Figures 11 a,b. Recanalization of the middle cerebral artery using BONNET system®: Complete right middle cerebral artery occlusion with collateral flow from the anterior cerebral artery territory (11a). Successful middle cerebral artery recanalization using the BONNET system® (11b).

Case Report 2

A 48-year-old male suffered from sudden left-sided hemiparesis, left facial nerve palsy and dysarthria (NIHSS 10 points). Findings on brain CT six hours after stroke onset were negative; CTA detected M1-MCA occlusion. CT perfusion did not detect any signs of definitive cerebral infarction. Digital subtractional angiography confirmed right MCA occlusion with collateral flow from the ACA territory (Figure 11a). Mechanical thrombectomy with BONNET device was performed 40 min after admission to hospital and immediate recanalization of MCA was achieved (Figure 11b). Patient's clinical status substantially improved immediately after the vessel reopening. Patient was without neurological deficit (mRS 0) at discharge.

pRESET Thrombectomy Retriever® (Phenox GmbH, Bochum, Germany)

The pRESET Thrombectomy Retriever® is another brand new thrombectomy device. The laser-cut and self-expanding Nitinol-System allows effective removal of clot material from 2 to 4 mm vessel diameter. An optimized cell design and a helically shaped slit enable a constant cell size, even in smaller vessels. The closed "ring" design at the proximal end of the system ensures a stable opening, less tapering when withdrawn and radial force on a steady level—Figure 12. The pRESET features an excentrical attachment to the insertion wire as well as X-ray visible markers at its proximal and distal ends. The System can be cleaned easily, and re-use in the same patient is possible. Its nominal size is 4 x 30 millimetres; it is delivered through 0.021" lumen microcatheter, and the technique of thrombus extraction is identical with previously described systems.

Case Report 3

A 51-year-old male was admitted to the hospital with sudden left-sided hemiparesis and dysartria (NIHSS 16 points). Chronic abuse of alcohol and nicotine were in patient history. CTA diagnosed right M1-MCA occlusion. Patient was on anticoagulation therapy due to prior cardiac failure, with INR 1.9 on admission. He was transferred to angiography, which confirmed MCA occlusion (Figure 13a). MCA recanalization was achieved with pRESET system four hours after onset of symptoms (Figure 13b). Follow-up rain CT revealed only small ischemic changes in right basal ganglia region. However, the clinical status has not improved (mRS 5 at discharge).

Current Studies In Stent Thrombectomy Devices

The recanalization rates clinical results of modern thrombectomy devices appear promising as the devices continue to evolve and become more operator-friendly. Baker et al. [34] screened citations for human studies of any design or case series or case reports of patients with an acute IS that evaluated a neurothrombectomy device and reported at least one clinical effectiveness outcome or harm. They identified 87 articles meeting eligibility criteria: 18 prospective single-group studies, seven noncomparative retrospective studies, and 62 case series or case reports. All prospective and retrospective studies provided data on successful recanalization. The recanalization rate widely varied (43 to 78% with the MERCI Retriever and 83 to 100% with the Penumbra System). SICH was evaluated in 16 studies and did not exceed 11%, and vessel perforation or dissection was between 0 and 7% and varied by device. Predictors of harm included older age, history of stroke, and higher baseline stroke severity scores, whereas successful recanalization was the sole predictor of good outcomes [34]. Unfortunately, the limitation of performed studies is missing evidence of a fragmentation, distal embolization, or relocation of the occlusive thrombus [35].

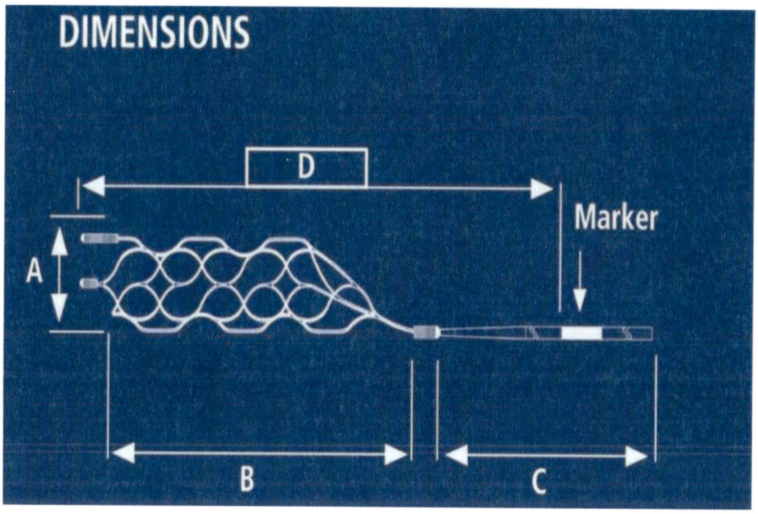

Figure 12. pRESET Thrombectomy Retriever® (Phenox GmbH, Bochum, Germany).

Three studies are underway in the United States and Europe to test retrievable stents in the treatment of acute IS. The Solitaire™ FR with the Intention for Thrombectomy (SWIFT) study is ongoing (recruitment completed) and will compare Solitaire FR with the Merci retriever in 200 patients. [36] The Trial and Cost Effectiveness Evaluation of IA Thrombectomy in acute IS (THRACE) study that will compare IVT with thrombectomy procedures using the Merci retriever, Penumbra system, Catch device (Balt Extrusion, Montmorency, France), and the Solitaire™ FB stent in 480 patients. The Thrombectomy Revascularization of Large Vessel Occlusions (TREVO 2) study was recently started in the United States and will compare the Trevo system versus the Merci retriever in the treatment of acute IS. Approximately 178 patients will be enrolled in the study [37].

The aim of an ongoing IMS-III trial is to investigate whether a combination of IVT and IAT is superior to standard IVT (standard dose of 0.9 mg/kg rt-PA). If the trombus is resolved, no additional intra-arterial therapy is administered. If the occlusion is still present, the additional intra-arterial treatment (max. 22 mg of rt-PA) will be administered. IAT might be combined with low-intensity ultrasound (US) via the EKOS® Micro-Infusion Catheter and thrombus-removal device as well. The clinical outcome is calculated by the mRS three months after the procedure. A total of 900 subjects will be enrolled in the study [38].

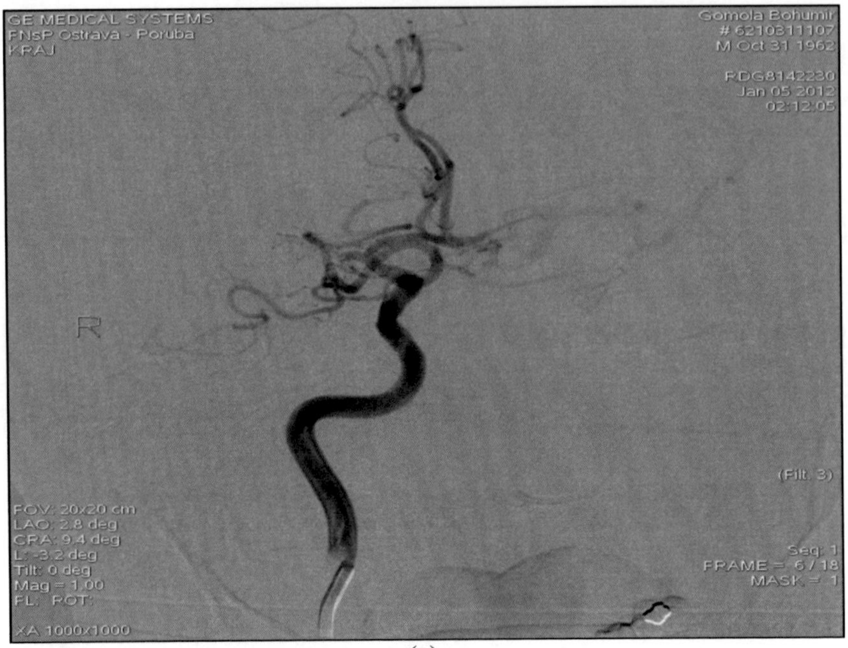

(a)

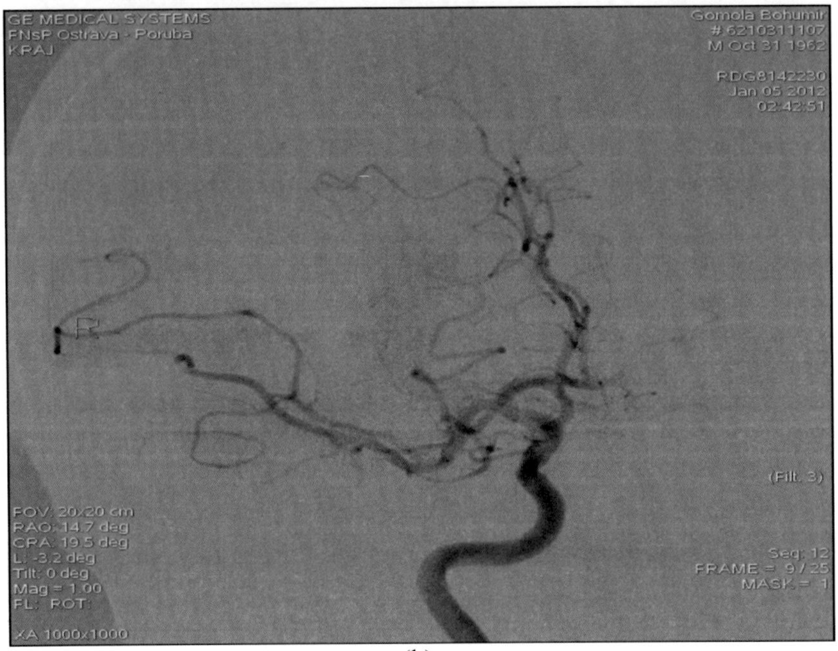

(b)

Figures 13 a,b. Recanalization of the middle cerebral artery using pRESET system®: Right middle cerebral artery occlusion (13a). Middle cerebral artery recanalization after two extractions using pRESET system® (13b).

The ongoing Mechanical Retrieval and Recanalization of Stroke Clots Using Embolectomy (MR-RESCUE) trial aids to evaluate the efficacy of the standard IVT in case of proximal main branch occlusion in the anterior circulation compared to the efficacy of mechanical thrombectomy (with MERCI or Penumbra) within eight hours after stroke onset [39].

In the DWI/PWI and CT perfusion assessment in the triage of wake-up and late presenting strokes undergoing neurointervention (DAWN) trial, patients with large artery occlusion are selected according to the magnetic resonance imaging (MRI) or CT perfusion images more than eight hours after stroke onset. The treatment is initiated between eight and 24 hours [40].

Direct Stent Placement

Intracranial self-expanding microstents have been used successfully as temporary or permanent endovascular bypass in the invasive management of acute IS. It has been performed most commonly as a rescue procedure to displace thrombus or following early reocclusion after successful fibrinolysis. Angioplasty with stenting was originally described in acute stroke for underlying atherosclerotic stenosis after successful fibrinolysis.

With this technique, the stent deployed at the point of vessel occlusion expands, displacing circumferentially the thrombus and allows flow restoration. The re-establishment of flow through the occlusion site promotes immediate dissipation of prothrombotic factors. At the same time, the restored arterial flow allows thrombolytic medications to be in contact with thrombotic material trapped within the mesh of the stent and against the arterial wall.

Various stents have been used over time to bridge the occlusion site. The first report of coronary balloon-mounted stent placement into the basilar artery was published in 1999, by Phatouros et al. [41]. These procedures were associated with high periprocedural major complication rates (up to 50%). Gradually, self-expanding stents came into use. In the past, stenting was used after failure of different recanalization approaches, i.e., angioplasty, IAT and thrombectomy with a snare device.

Self-expandable stents were approved for vessel remodeling in the treatment of cerebral aneurysms and intracranial atherosclerotic disease. The Enterprise stent (Cordis Neurovascular, Miami Lakes, FL, US), the Neuroform system (Stryker, Natick, MA, US), and the Leo stent (Balt Extrusion, Montmorency, France) are devices introduced for stent-assisted coiling of wide-neck aneurysms. The latter stent is not marketed in the United States. The Wingspan system (Stryker, Natick, MA, US) was approved for treatment of intracranial atherosclerosis. Both the Neuroform and Wingspan stents have an open-cell design, whereas the Enterprise and Leo stents are closed-cell design—Figure 14. [42] The closed-cell design allows resheathing of the stent after partial deployment (70% for Enterprise and 90% for Leo).

These devices have been used off-label in the treatment of acute IS. The concept of flow restoration without clot removal has gained attention as other recanalization approaches that focus their strategy in thrombectomy have failed.

Published Studies

Fitzsimmons and Nelson reported one of the first cases of cerebral revascularization with deployment of a self-expansible stent. [43] A Neuroform stent was deployed in an occluded left MCA after the IA infusion of a glycoprotein (GP) IIb/IIIa inhibitor failed to recanalize the vessel. Multiple reports have followed, especially from the group lead by Levy et al. [44], who have pioneered the use of self-expansible stents in the treatment of acute IS. In 2007, they reported a 100% successful deployment of stents (16 Neuroform and three Wingspan stents) in the target occlusion, achieving a recanalization TIMI score 2 – 3 in 79% of lesions. Four (22%) patients had a mRS ≤ 3 at three months and two (11%) patients suffered SICH.

Most of the studies published to date have been retrospective single-center reports with sample sizes ranging between nine and 20 patients [45-49]. Although these cohorts are small, recanalization rates of 92 and 100% have been reported in cases where other thrombectomy devices have failed [46,47,49]. Another two small studies reported recanalization rates with cerebral angioplasty 60 to 90% and good outcomes (mRS 0 – 2 or NIHSS ≤ 4) between 36 and 74% [50,51]. Jovin reported successful recanalization in 23 out of the 25 patients, one SICH and one carotid dissection. [52]

The recently reported preliminary data of a prospective Stent-Assisted Recanalization in acute IS (SARIS) study of first 20 patients with acute IS showed the successful recanalization (TIMI grade 2/3) in 100% of cases with a 5% rate of SICH. [53] A six-month follow-up of the SARIS trial found mRS ≤ 2 in 55% of patients with a mortality rate of 35%. None of the patients had in-stent restenosis and all had TIMI-3 flow in angiographic follow-up [54].

There is growing experience with intracranial stenting in the acute IS setting, which has brought encouraging findings. Stenting is technically feasible, as reported up to 100% successful deployment rate of different studies. Acute in-stent thrombosis is rare, and different treatment strategies may be used to achieve stent recanalization: intra-arterial administration of GP IIb/IIIa inhibitors or stent resheathing. Enterprise stents appear to have better navigability than the Wingspan and Neuroform stents, especially in acute IS patients who generally have a tortuous anatomy with atherosclerotic changes. Self-expanding stents have enough radial force to recanalize occluded arteries. Angiographic outcomes have improved since the first series published by Levy et al. achieving TIMI 2/3 flow in more than 90% of lesions. Antiplatelet agents such as aspirin and clopidogrel or GP IIb/IIIa inhibitors should be administered prior to stent deployment to avoid acute in-stent thrombosis. However, this may lead to SICH if thrombolytic agents have been previously administered.

Intracranial stenting in acute IS patients certainly has many potential drawbacks. Permanent stent deployment in the setting of acute IS requires platelet inhibition to reduce the possibility of in-stent thrombosis. Intra-procedural administration of GP IIb/IIIa inhibitors or inhibitors of platelet function (Anopyrin®, Cardegic®) may increase the risk of hemorrhagic transformation. Furthermore, dual antiplatelet therapy is continued for at least the initial three months after the procedure. This is particularly worrisome in patients who already have been treated with IVT and/or IAT. Stent placement in acute IS is a permanent implant to resolve a temporary occlusion that may be caused by an embolus. Stent deployment may over time result in delayed in-stent stenosis. With expansion of the stent, the thrombus material may be pushed into perforating arteries. This phenomenon, described as "snow-plowing," may explain strokes in perforator territories once the main artery has been recanalized and may pose another drawback of this technique.

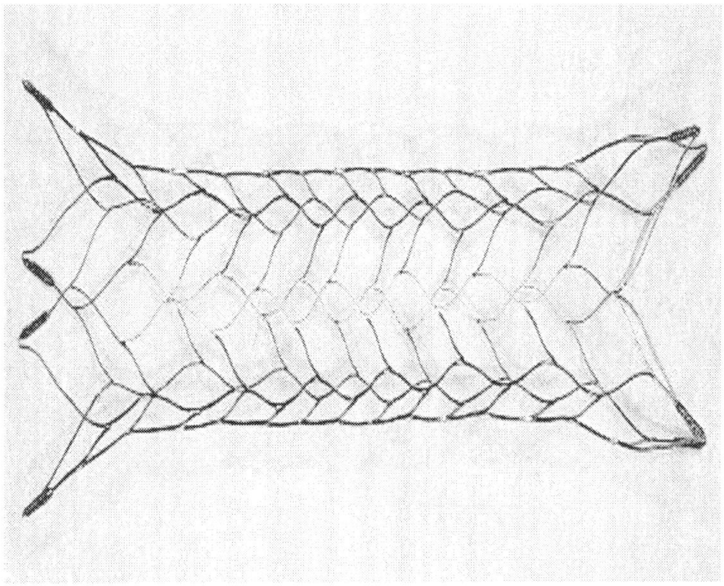

Figure 14. Enterprise stent (Cordis Neurovascular, Miami Lakes, FL, US).

Case Report 4

A 61-year-old female suffered from sudden loss of consciousness, dysartria and right-sided hemiparesis (NIHSS 15 points). Only hypercholesterolemia was in medical history. CTA revealed the occlusion of the left M1-MCA. Patient was treated with IVT (80 mg of rt-PA) 115 minutes after stroke onset without improvement of the clinical status. Persistent occlusion of the MCA was detected on angiography (Figure 15a). Left MCA was recanalized using cerebral percutaneous angioplasty with intracranial stent implantation three hours and 50 minutes after symptoms onset (Figure 15b). Follow-up brain CT detected infarction in the left basal ganglia. On discharge, patient presented with severe right-sided central hemiparesis and global aphasia (mRS 5).

Case Report 5

A 77-year-old male suffered from vertigo and vomiting, gradual progression of dysartria and left-sided hemiparesis. Arterial hypertension and diabetes mellitus were in medical history. Severe basilar stenosis was detected on CTA performed two hours and 50 minutes after stroke onset. Upon transfer to angiography, tachypnoe, worsening of consciousness and quadriparesis evolved. Patient was intubated and angiography detected left vertebral artery stenosis and basilar artery occlusion (Figure 16a). Attempt to recanalize the occlusion was undertaken 3.5 hours after onset of symptoms. However, the procedure failed with contrast media paravasation at the site of vertebral intradural segment dissection caused by microwire (Figure 16b). Follow-up CT scan revealed ischemic changes in the pons and cerebellum and subarachnoid bleeding in posterior fossa. Patient was discharged in a poor clinical state (mRS 5).

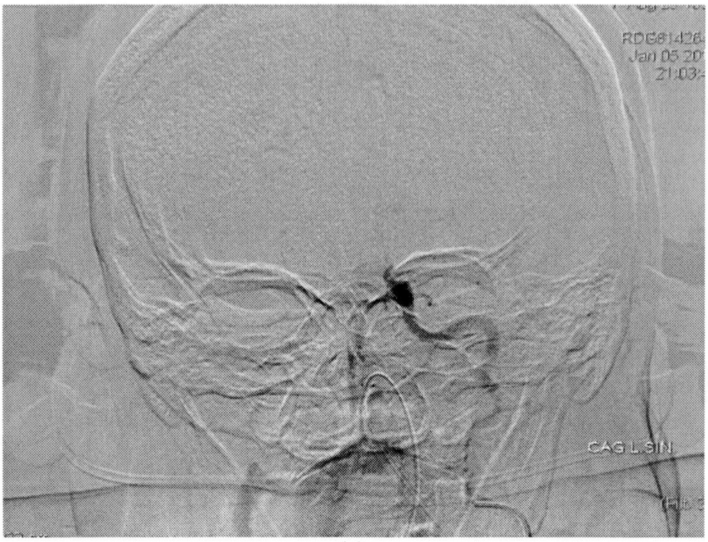

(a)

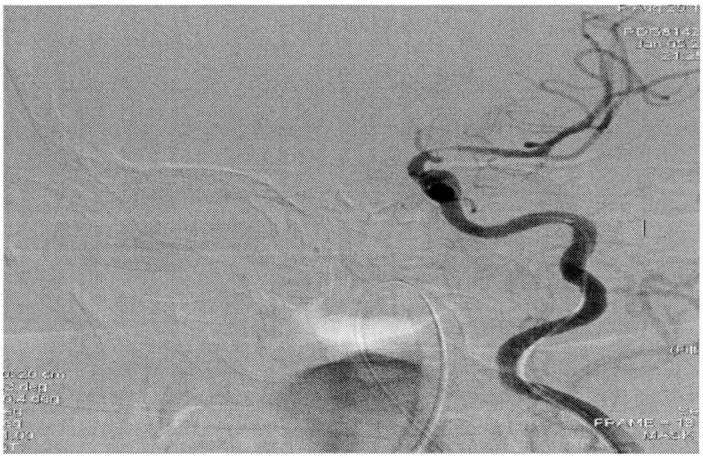

(b)

Figures 15 a,b. Recanalization of the distal occlusion of the internal carotid artery and the middle cerebral artery using cerebral percutaneous angioplasty and stenting: Distal occlusion of the internal carotid artery demonstrated on angiography (15a). Recanalization of the internal carotid artery and the middle cerebral artery after direct intracranial stent deployment (15b).

Endovascular Sono-Lysis—EkoSonic™ Endovascular System (EKOS Corporation, Bothell, WA, US)

Although the complex effect of ultrasound on the acceleration of thrombus lysis is not yet fully understood, it is assumed that the ultrasonic waves accelerate enzymatic fibrinolysis by primarily non-thermal mechanisms—increasing the transport of fibrinolytic agents into the thrombus by mechanical disruption of its structure [55], direct activation of fibrinolytic enzymes, either mechanical breaking of the complex molecules, in which fibrinolytic enzymes are inactivated by binding to their inhibitors, or irritation of the endothelium with increased production of fibrinolytic enzymes [56,57], transient peripheral (capillary) vasodilatation caused probably by increased production of nitrite oxide in the endothelium [58,59]. Radiation force and acoustic cavitation are the next possible and discussed mechanical effects of ultrasound [60].

There are two possibilities for sono-lysis application—transcranial approach through intact skull or intravascular approach.

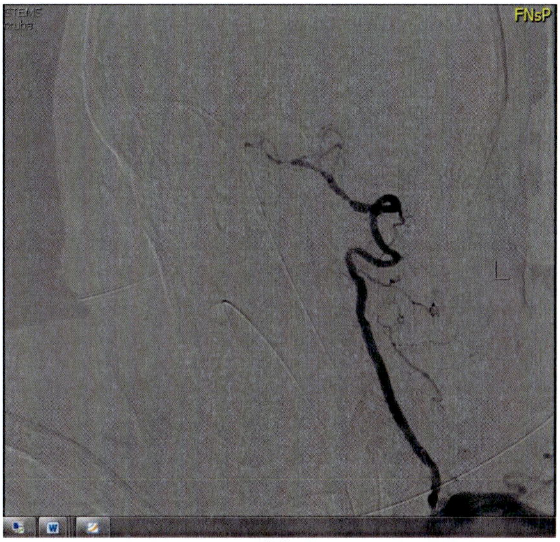

(a)

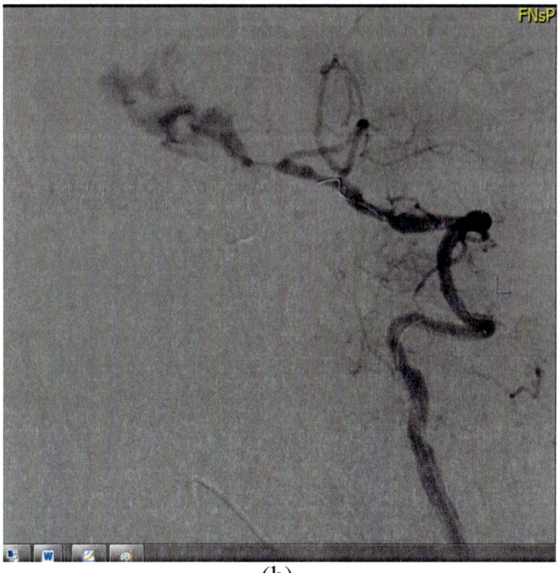

(b)

Figures 16 a,b. Complications during recanalization of the basilar artery occlusion: Diffuse left vertebral artery atherosclerotic lesions with severe stenosis of V3-segment of left vertebral artery and artery occlusion distal to posterior inferior cerebellar artery origin (16a). Severe paravasation after iatrogenic vertebral dissection caused by microwire passage (16b).

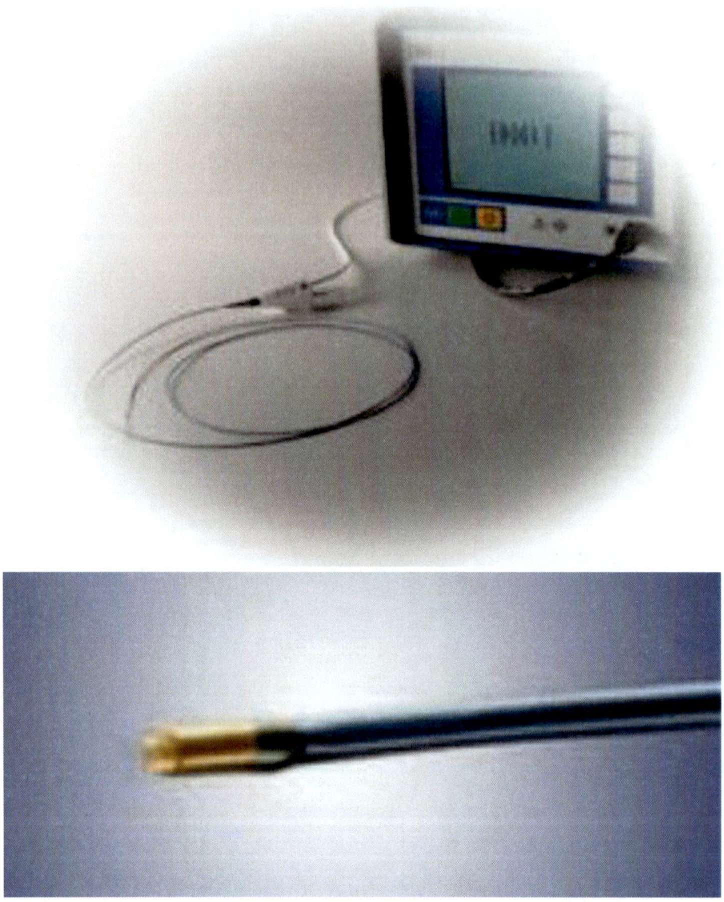

(a)

(b)

Figure 17 a,b. EkoSonic™ Endovascular System (EKOS Corporation, Bothell, WA, US).

The EkoSonic™ Endovascular System (EKOS Corporation, Bothell, WA, US) is intended for targeted local drug delivery including rt-PA where non-cavitational, high–frequency, low-power microsonic energy allows better penetration and attachment of a thrombolytic agent into the thrombus, resulting in faster lysis and a vessel recanalization, as was proved by manufacturer in in vitro testing—Figure 17 a,b. The system consists of a single-use EKOS MicroLys US infusion catheter intended either for neurovascular interventions EkoSonicSV™ (3F/150 cm catheter inserted over a 0.014" wire) or for peripheral procedures EkoSonic™ (over a 0.035" wire). The outer diameter of the catheter is rather small and can be easily introduced through 6F guiding catheter, which is advantageous compared to some other devices. The catheters have a hollow end-hole infusion lumen incorporating cylindrical piezo transducer at its tip, which converts high-frequency energy into ultrasound waves. In EkoSonicSV™, the transducer power output is 0.45 W at a frequency of 1.4 – 1.9 MHz. The energy deployment causes non-cavitational fibrin strands thinning, loosens up the fibrin matrix and thus increases the availability of plasminogen activation receptor sites for plasminogen/plasmin binding. Bound plasminogen/plasmin is then protected from alfa2-antiplasmin inhibition. According to the manufacturer's data, thrombus exposed to ultrasonic pressure absorbed 48% more rt-PA in one hour than in conventional catheter local drug delivery. The clot lysis is four times faster than with the conventional catheter-directed thrombolysis alone in manufacturer in-vitro experiments. It has been suggested that EkoSonicSV™ dissolves a clot more homogenously and completely with minimal residual thrombi and a low risk of distal embolism by dislocated clot fragments. There is a thermoreceptor placed at the catheter tip for continuous intraprocedural temperature monitoring. Increase in temperature may indicate vessel patency or local accumulation of energy in the clot and surrounding tissues by ultrasound waves. Since the output power and catheter temperature are continuously monitored, this therapy poses a low risk of the vessel wall and surrounding tissue damage and impairment. Due to these reasons, the vessel patency is reached faster with the smaller total doses of thrombolytic agents when compared to standard thrombolysis.

The other part of the system is the central unit, which generates the specific frequency energy and monitors the output power, along with the temperature of the catheter tip—Figure 17 a,b.

Published Studies

A phase I trial reported preliminary results of treatment using the EkoSonicSV™ system in 14 patients with 60% recanalization at 60 minutes, despite treatment of large clot burdens in some patients [61]. The device was tested again in the Interventional Management of Stroke (IMS) II with promising results [62]. Complete recanalization was achieved within 60 and 120 minutes in 12 (41%) and 20 (68.9%) patients, respectively. The authors compared their results with the findings from the IMS-1 clinical trial. They concluded that recanalization has been achieved in seven (30.4%) of the 23 control patients from the IMS-1 trial. Pooled analysis based on the results of these two studies showed complete recanalization in 120 minutes in 68.9% of patients in the EkoSonic™ catheter sonography group compared with 53.3% of patients treated by standard microcatheter infusion technique. Due to these promising results, acute stroke in NINDS rt-PA-funded IMS III trial globally, which is currently enrolling at 60 stroke centers worldwide [38]. Furthermore, the SICH occurred in 8/81 (9.9%) subjects in the IMS-II, including 1/26 (3.8%) patients treated with IV rt-PA alone and one in a sonography microcatheter–treated subject without the use of sonography. No direct vessel perforation, primary subarachnoid hemorrhage, or intracranial dissection was documented in the treated subjects.

According to the authors' experiences, the EkoSonic™ catheter is easy to introduce despite the non-flexible sonography transducer located at its distal tip [63]. The authors did not encounter any detectable distal embolization potentially resulting from device manipulation. However, the risk of distal embolization was an issue in Janjua's study [64]. Although the distal emboli were observed in their study, this situation did not have any significant clinical consequences. On the other hand, distal embolisation was not detected in other studies [65,66]. The clot resolution time in patients presented by the authors (vessel patency in 35 minutes) was much quicker than in the IMS-2 study, where complete resolution of a clot was achieved after one hour in 41.1% of patients. One may speculate that such a promising result may be caused by the fresh (noncrossed-linked) nature of the clot.

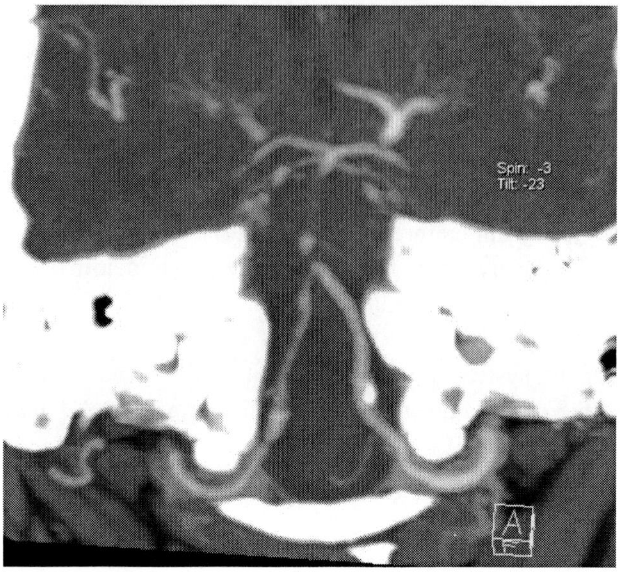

(a)

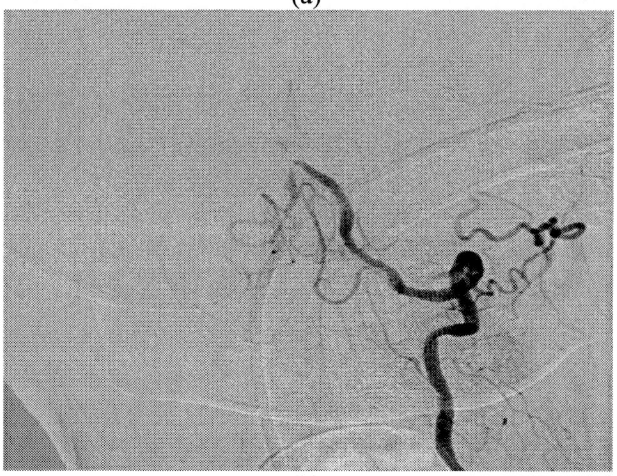

(b)

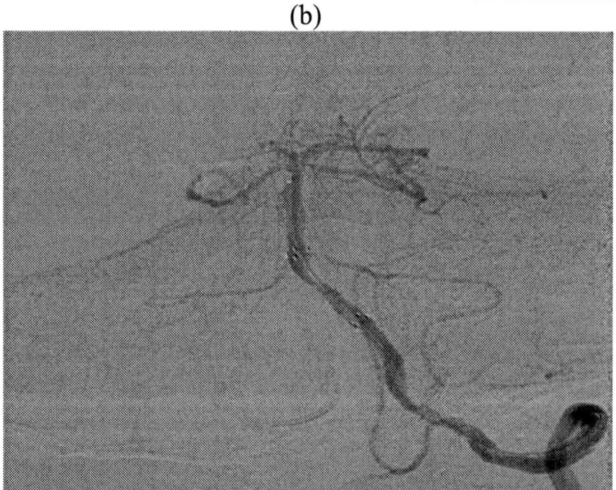

(c)

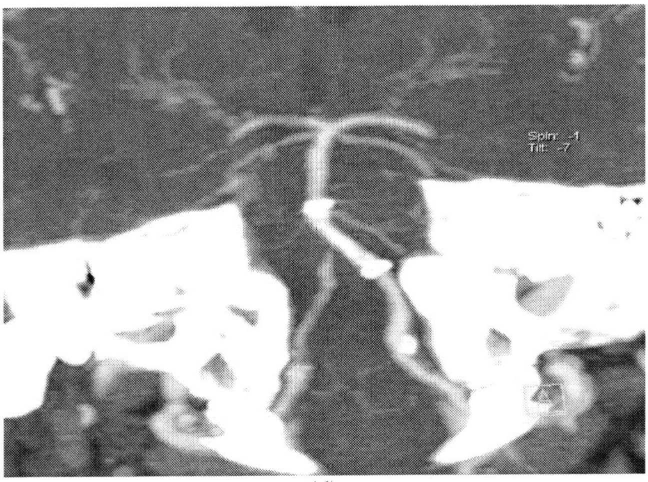

(d)

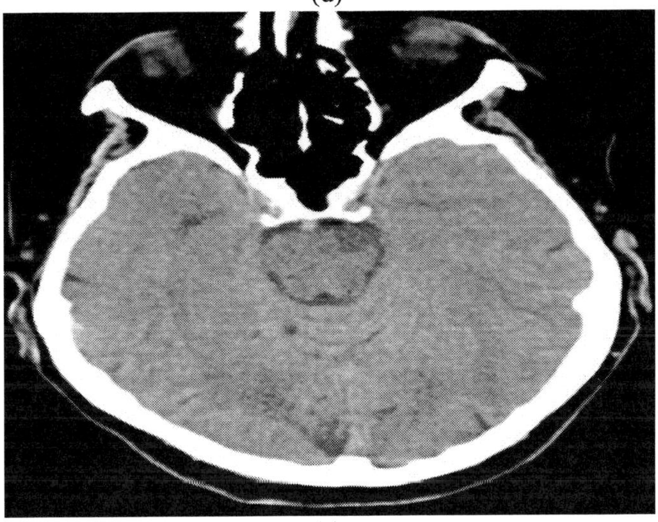

(e)

Figures 18a-e. Recanalization of the basilar artery using intravascular sonolysis by EkoSonic™ Endovascular System. CT angiography detected severe proximal basilar artery stenosis in junction of vertebral arteries and occlusion of distal part of basilar artery; the tip of basilar artery and posterior cerebral arteries are perfused through the posterior communicating arteries collateral blood flow (18a). Angiographic finding of basilar artery occussion via the left vertebral artery (18b). Cerebral percutaneous transluminal angioplasty with Wingspan stent 3,5 x 15 insertion to the proximal basilar artery stenosis and EkoSonic™ microcatheter sonolysis 35 minutes after rt-PA administration (18c). Follow-up CT angiography (maximum intensity projection—MIP) showed patent basilar artery with stent and normal filling of bilateral anterior inferior cerebellar artery, superior cerebellar artery and posterior cerebrellar artery. Severe stenosis of the right vertebral artery is apparent (18d). CT scan at day two showed infarctions in the left pons and in the right posterior cerebral artery territory - calcarine artery feeding territory (18e).

Case Report 6

A 60-year-old female was admitted to a local hospital with right humeral neck fracture. Four hours later, while being on a conservative therapy regime, she was suddenly unable to speak, and right-sided hemiplegia was diagnosed (NIHSS 19 points). Arterial hypertension, hypercholesterolemia, ischemic heart disease with coronary bypass and diabetes mellitus were in medical history. The immediate CT scan was negative for signs of ischemia and haemorrhage. CTA showed severe stenosis of both vertebral arteries at the junction level and basilar artery occlusion (Figure 18a). CT perfusion scans revealed prolonged time to peak value in the posterior fossa structures and occipital lobes of the brain. No substantial changes in blood volume and blood flow parameters were observed. The patient was transferred to angiography, which confirmed findings of basilar artery occusion via the left vertebral artery. Intracranial stent Wingspan 3.5/20 mm (Boston Scientific, Fremont, CA, USA) was placed into the proximal basilar artery stenosis (Figure 18c). Thereafter, the EkoSonic™ catheter insonation was performed (Figure 18c) and completed successful basilar artery recanalization eight hours after stroke onset was achieved (Figure 18d). Follow-up CT revealed small brainstem infarction (Figure 18e). At discharge, residual dysartria and right-sided central hemiparesis persisted (mRS 4).

Other Experimental Devices EPAR®—Endovascular Photoacoustic Recanalization (Endovasix Inc., Belmont, CA, US)

EPAR® is a mechanical clot fragmentation device based on laser technology (endovascular photo-acoustic reanalization—EPAR®). This device consists of three French hydrophilically coated microcatheters with five windows at its tip, each of them with one optic fiber. The photonic energy, delivered at a rate of 1,000 optic pulses per second, is converted into acoustic energy at the fiberoptic tip of the catheter. This in turn creates micro-cavitation bubbles. The cavitation pockets undergo expansion and subsequent collapse and should create suction of the thrombus through the lateral windows into the catheter tip. Inside the tip, the clot is emulsified, and the tip contents are discharged as subcapillary-size particles (in vitro: 1 to 10 μm). This system is intended as fast clot emulsifier rather than laser-ablation device. The main objective is to provoke mechanical thrombolysis and reduce the amount of pharmacological thrombolytics needed.

Studies

Thirty-four patients (median NIHSS 19) were enrolled in the study published by Berlis et al. [67]. Ten patients had ICA occlusion, 12 patients MCA occlusion, 11 patients vertebrobasilar occlusion, and one patient posterior cerebral artery occlusion. The overall recanalization rate was 41.1%. Complete EPAR® treatment was possible in 18 patients (median NIHSS 18), with vessel recanalization achieved in 11 patients (61.1%) after EPAR. The average time of procedure was 9.65 minutes. Incomplete EPAR® treatment (16/34, median NIHSS 19) was defined as intention to treat with EPAR® and that the EPAR® microcatheter entered the patient. Additional treatment with IA application of rt-PA was used in 13 patients. An adverse event associated with the use of the device occurred in one patient. SICH occurred in two patients (5.9%). The mortality rate was 38.2%. Unfortunately, this device is not marketed any longer.

Revive™ SE Blood Clot Retrieval® (Codman and Shurtleff, Inc., Johnson and Johnson Company, Raynham, MA, US)

Revive™ SE® is intended as a blood clot retrieval and removal device. Its self-expanding nitinol basket should act as a temporary bypass across the occlusion and subsequently can be used for thrombus removal. It is introduced via a microcatheter directly into or beyond the lesion and can be redeployed several times. It is designed as a closed distal end basket that should engage the clot effectively and prevent it from distal embolisation.

The company received CE Mark approval for the Revive™ SE® in February 2011. The device is not approved for distribution in the United States.

Pilot results of ten patients with acute large vessel occlusions treated with the Revive device was published by Rohde at al. Vessel recanalization (TICI 2b or 3) was successful in all patients without device-related complications. After one month, six patients had a clinical improvement of >8 points or an NIHSS 0 – 1; three patients died. SICH occurred in two patients. [68]

This device is going to be investigated in a single-arm German study named RIVER I (Reperfuse Ischemic Vessels with Endovascular Recanalization). The patients will be screened before the procedure with MRI imaging.

Penumbra Separator™ 3d® (Penumbra, Alameda, CA, US)

Penumbra Separator™ 3D® is a brand new product that was introduced in January 2012, dedicated for thrombus retrieval in acute stroke patients. Its design resembles complex 3D "basket." Its inner struts and complex design is aimed at firm thrombus engagement and reliable retraction. Like other stentrievers, it is deployed into the occluded vessel segment with micocatheter, and retrieval is bolstered by active aspiration via guiding catheter.

At ABC-WIN Seminar, Prof. M. Knauth presented the European evaluation data on Separator 3D [69]. The first preliminary data from six European centers with this new device showed an approximately 90% successful recanalizations and good deliverability even in tortuous vessels.

Mindframe Capture LP® (Mindframe Inc., Irvine, CA, US)

MindFrame capture LP® is another stent-like device aimed at temporary by-pass reopening of the occluded vessels and effective thrombectomy—Figure 19.

Its advantage is compatibility with 10/14 microcatheters with inner diameter from 0.0165 inch. It received an CE mark in August 2011, and first results in treating stroke patients were presented by Tommy Andersson, MD, PhD, Department of Neuroradiology, Karolinska University Hospital, Stockholm, who stated that this devices allowed good ability to access thrombus through tortuous blood vessel anatomies and showed fair recanalizations rate (personal communications).

Acandis APERIO® System (Acandis Gmbh and Co. KG, Pforzheim, Germany)

Acandis APERIO® System is a self-expanding stent-like clot retrieval system that can be deployed through 0.027" inner lumen microcatheter and bolsters superb trackability and good thrombus removal rate of about 80%—Figure 20. No published data are available so far.

Possis Angiojet System® (Possis Medical, Minneapolis, MN, US)

This is a five-Frech system based on rheolytic thrombectomy effect, caused by fast high-pressure saline jets that creates distal Venturi suction and leads to clot fragmentation and aspiration. First case reports of ICA recanalization procedures with this device were published [70].

Latis Laser Device® (Spectanetics, Colorado Springs, CO, US)

This is also a microcatheter with laser at its tip. Contrast media injection was used for energy transfer from the catheter into the thrombus. The safety and feasibility study was stopped after enrollment of only 12 patients, since there were difficulties in deployment of the catheter to the level of occlusion. This device is not marketed any longer.

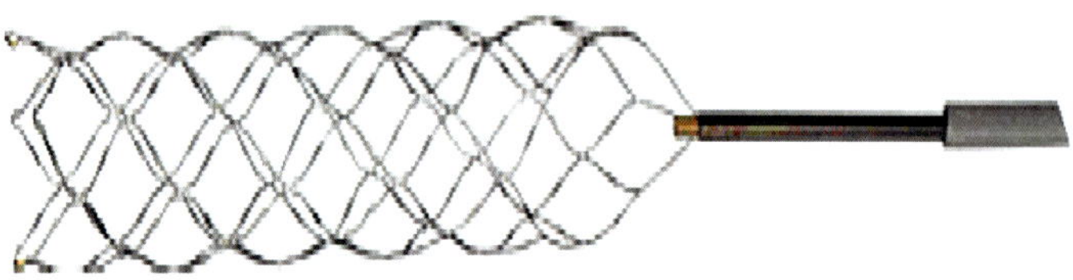

Figure 19. Mindframe capture LP®.

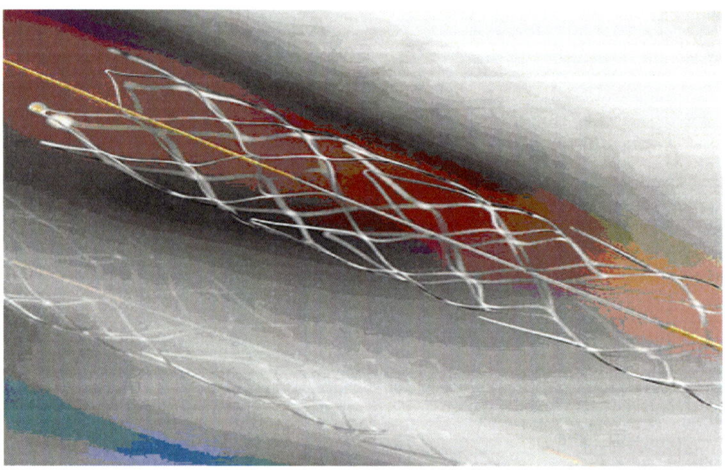

Figure 20. Acandis APERIO System®.

Amplatz Goose-Neck Microsnare® (Ev3 Medical, Plymouth, MN, US)

The system consists of microcatheter, snare and rotator. The microsnare is constructed of a nitinol cable and gold plated tungsten loop. This nitinol snare was used for clot retrieval in cases of solid thrombus with firm consistency. In cases of soft thrombus, multiple passes of the snare through the thrombus were used to disrupt its structure.

Attracter-18™ (Boston Scientific/Target Therapeutics, Fremont, CA, US)

Another so called "goose-neck" snare, primarily developed to retrieve dislodged coils during cerebral aneurysm coiling procedure. Both these devices were not originally intended for thrombectomy in IS patients.

Neuronet™ Guidant Device® (Guidant Corp, Temecula, CA, US)

Neuronet is a self-expanding basket introduced distally to a clot by a microcatheter. After if unfolds, it is retracted back into the thrombus and should pull the thrombus into the micro catheter.

In-Time™ Retrieval Device® (Boston Scientific, Boston, MA, US)

The principle of clot removal is the same as in the Neuronet Guidant device.

Interventional Procedure Technique

In the authors' department, most of the procedures are performed under conscious sedation or under general anesthesia. Common femoral artery is the most common access site. In a few patients, in whom iliac arteries were occluded, the recanalization procedure was performed via brachial access. Mostly 6F or 8F sheath and 4F diagnostic catheters introduced over hydrophilic wires are used. As the first step, brain supplying vessels angiography is performed to evaluate the site of occlusion and extent of collateral supply. When endovascular recanalization is indicated, the 6F or 8F guiding catheter is inserted into the ICA or the vertebral artery. Subsequently, microcatheter supported by microwire sized 0,010" to 0,018" is inserted into the occlusion site. The authors try to navigate the microcatheter past the occlusion site to verify the lengths of the occlusion and to check if distal embolization is present. It is an absolutely duty to perform control microcatheter angiography after passing the occlusion to confirm the intraluminal position of the catheter and to exclude any vessel dissection or perforation. Having done this, the decision as to which of the recanalization methods will be engaged for this particular case is made. This requires exchange of the catheter for the particular dedicated device. The interventionalist has to have more endovascular devices in store, since every patient is unique and the recanalization must be well tailored for the particular situation. Usually, 50 I.U. per kilogram (max. 3000 I.U.) of Heparin® are administered at the beginning of the procedure to prevent clot formation on introduced equipment. Furthermore, heparinized saline is used to continually flush all coaxial systems. Although some authors discourage the use of Heparin®, the authors have not encountered any substantial bleeding into the ischemic brain tissue over the past six years.

To conclude, the way of microcatheter introduction into intracranial vessels is standardized at the authors' institution and does not differ much between various intracranial endovascular procedures performed with different devices.

After successful artery reopening, any possible residual restenosis (or residual stenosis) at the original occlusion site should be precisely evaluated and treated if needed. The other very important issue is to evaluate is distal arteries patency. Any distal embolization or residual occlusion has to be excluded. If eligible, patients with reocclusion are treated with IA rt-PA administration. Last, but not least, the proximal parts of the brain supplying vessels should be evaluated and treated if needed.

Conclusion

Early recanalization is associated with a significantly higher chance of independency after 90 days, with a significant reduction of mortality. In addition to pharmacological methods (IVT and IAT), mechanical neuro-interventional methods are intensively tested and introduced into clinical practice. Results of first studies showed safety and efficacy of various devices with increasing recanalization rate and relative low number of peri-procedural complications and SICH. However, clinical benefit for acute stroke patients has to be confirmed in prospective studies.

Acknowledgment

Partially supported by the grants from the Internal Grant Agency of Ministry of Health of Czech Republic number NT/11386-5/2010 and NT/11046-6/2010.

References

[1] Feigin, VL; Lawes, CM; Bennett, DA; Anderson, CS. Stroke epidemiology: a review of population-based studies of incidence, prevalence, and case-fatality in the late 20th century. *Lancet Neurol*, 2003, 2, 43-53.

[2] Rosamond, W; Flegal, K; Furie, K; Go, A; Greenlund, K; Haase, N; Hailpern, SM; Ho, M; Howard, V; Kissela, B; Kittner, S; Lloyd-Jones, D; McDermott, M; Meigs, J; Moy, C; Nichol, G; O'Donnell, C; Roger, V; Sorlie, P; Steinberger, J; Thom, T; Wilson, M; Hong, Y. Heart disease and stroke statistics - 2008 update: a report from the American Heart Association Statistics Committee and Stroke Statistics Subcommittee. Circulation, 2008, 117, e25-146.

[3] Fieschi, C; Argentino, C; Lenzi, GL; Sacchetti, ML; Toni, D; Bozzao, L. Clinical and instrumentalevaluation of patients with ischemic stroke within the first six hours. *J Neurol Sci,* 1989, 91, 311-321.

[4] van der Worp, HB; van Gijn, J. Clinical practice. Acute ischemic stroke. *N Engl J Med*, 2007, 357, 572-579.

[5] Rha, JH; Saver, JL. The impact of recanalization on ischemic stroke outcome: a meta-analysis. *Stroke*, 2007, 38, 967-73.

[6] Blakeley, JO; Llinas, RH. Thrombolytic therapy for acute ischemic stroke. *J Neurol Sci*, 2007, 261, 55-62.

[7] Brott, T; Bogousslavsky, J. Treatment of acute ischemic stroke. *N Engl J Med*, 2000, 343, 710-722.

[8] The National Institute of Neurological Disorders and Stroke rt-PA Stroke Study Group Tissue plasminogen activator for acute ischemic stroke. *N Engl J Med*, 1995, 333, 1581-1587.

[9] Smith, WS; Sung, G; Starkman, S; Saver, JL; Kidwell, CS; Gobin, YP; Lutsep, HL; Nesbit, GM; Grobelny, T; Rymer, MM; Silverman, IE; Higashida, RT; Budzik, RF; Marks, MP; MERCI Trial Investigators. Safety and efficacy of mechanical embolectomy in acute ischemic stroke: results of the MERCI trial. *Stroke*, 2005, 36, 1432-1440.

[10] Chopko, BW; Kerber, C; Wong, W; Georgy, B. Transcatheter snare removal of acute middle cerebral artery thromboembolism: technical case report. *Neurosurgery*, 2000, 46, 1529-1531.

[11] Kerber, CW; Barr, JD; Berger, RM; Chopko, BW. Snare retrieval of intracranial thrombus in patients with acute stroke. *J Vasc Interv Radiol* 2002, 13, 1269-1274.

[12] Fourie, P; Duncan, IC. Microsnare-assisted mechanical removal of intraprocedural distal middle cerebral arterial thromboembolism. *Am J Neuroradiol*, 2003, 24, 630-632.

[13] Schumacher, HC; Meyers, PM; Yavagal, DR; Harel, NY; Elkind, MS; Mohr, JP; Pile-Spellman, J. Endovascular mechanical thrombectomy of an occluded superior division branch of the left MCA for acute cardioembolic stroke. *Cardiovasc Intervent Radiol*, 2003, 26, 305-308.

[14] Baker, WL; Colby, JA; Tongbram, V; Talati, RA; Silverman, IE; White, CM; Kluger, J; Coleman, CI. Neurothrombectomy Devices for Treatment of Acute Ischemic Stroke. Executive Summary. Effective Health Care Program, 2011, 7, ES1-ES9.

[15] Smith, WS; for the Multi MERCI Investigators. Safety of Mechanical Thrombectomy and Intravenous Tissue Plasminogen Activator in Acute Ischemic Stroke. Results of the Multi Mechanical Embolus Removal in Cerebral Ischemia (MERCI) Trial, Part I. *Am J Neuroradiol*, 2006, 27, 1177–1182.

[16] Smith, WS; Sung, G; Saver, J; Budzik, R; Duckwiler, G; Liebeskind, DS; Lutsep, HL; Rymer, MM; Higashida, RT; Starkman, S; Gobin, YP; for the Multi MERCI Investigators Mechanical Thrombectomy for Acute Ischemic Stroke Final Results of the Multi MERCI Trial. *Stroke*, 2008, 39, 1205-1212.

[17] Nogueira, RG; Smith, WS; Sung, G; Duckwiler, G; Walker, G; Roberts, R; Saver, JL; Liebeskind, DS; MERCI and Multi MERCI Writing Committee. Effect of time to reperfusion on clinical outcome of anterior circulation strokes treated with thrombectomy: pooled analysis of the MERCI and Multi MERCI trials. *Stroke*, 2011, 42, 3144-3149.

[18] Nogueira, RG; Liebeskind, DS; Sung, G; Duckwiler, G; Smith, WS; on Behalf of the MERCI; and Multi MERCI Writing Committee. Predictors of Good Clinical Outcomes, Mortality, and Successful Revascularization in Patients With Acute Ischemic Stroke Undergoing Thrombectomy Pooled Analysis of the Mechanical Embolus Removal in Cerebral Ischemia (MERCI) and Multi MERCI Trials. *Stroke*, 2009, 40, 3777-3783.

[19] Josephson, SA; Saver, JL; Smith, WS; Merci and Multi Merci Investigators. Comparison of mechanical embolectomy and intra-arterial thrombolysis in acute ischemic stroke within the MCA: MERCI and Multi MERCI compared to PROACT II. *Neurocrit Care*, 2009, 10, 43-49.

[20] Shi, Z-S; Loh, Y; Walker, G; Duckwiler, GR; for the MERCI and Multi-MERCI Investigators. Occlusions versus Secondary Division Occlusions After Mechanical Thrombectomy Pooled Anysis of the Mechanical Embolus Removal in Cerebral Ischemia (MERCI) and Multi MERCI Trials. *Stroke*, 2010, 41, 953-960.

[21] Flint, AC; Duckwiler, GR; Budzik, RF; Liebeskind, DS; Smith, WS; for the MERCI and Multi MERCI Writing Committee Mechanical Thrombectomy of Intracranial Internal Carotid Occlusion Pooled Results of the MERCI and Multi MERCI Part I Trials. *Stroke*, 2007, 38, 1274-1280.

[22] Lutsep, HL; Rymer, MM; Nesbit, GM. Vertebrobasilar revascularization rates and outcomes in the MERCI and multi-MERCI trials. *J Stroke Cerebrovasc Dis*, 2008, 17, 55-57.

[23] The Penumbra Pivotal Stroke Trial: safety and effectiveness of a new generation of mechanical devices for clot removal in intracranial large vessel occlusive disease. *Stroke*, 2009, 40, 2761–2768.

[24] Saver, JL; Liebeskind, DS; Nogueira, RG; Jahan, R. Need to clarify Thrombolysis In Myocardial Ischemia (TIMI) scale scoring method in the Penumbra Pivotal Stroke Trial. *Stroke*, 2010, 41, e115–e116.

[25] Grunwald, IQ; Wakhloo, AK; Walter, S. Endovascular Stroke Treatment Today. *Am J Neuroradiol*, 2011, 32, 238–43.

[26] Castaño, C; Dorado, L; Guerrero, C; Millan, M; Gomis, M; Perez de la Ossa, N; Castellanos, M; García, MR; Domenech, S; Dávalos, A. Mechanical thrombectomy with the Solitaire AB device in large artery occlusions of the anterior circulation: a pilot study. *Stroke*, 2010, 41, 1836-1840.

[27] Machi, P; Costalat, V; Lobotesis, K; Lima Maldonado, I; Vendrell, JF; Riquelme, C; Bonafe, A. Solitaire FR thrombectomy system: immediate results in 56 consecutive acute ischemic stroke patients. *J Neurointerv Surg*, 2012, 4, 62-66.

[28] Roth, C; Papanagiotou, P; Behnke, S; Walter, S; Haass, A; Becker, C; Fassbender, K; Politi, M; Körner, H; Romann, MS; Reith, W. Stent-assisted mechanical recanalization for treatment of acute intracerebral artery occlusions. *Stroke*, 2010, 41, 2559-2567.

[29] Seifert, M; Ahlbrecht, A; Dohmen, C; Spuentrup, E; Moeller-Hartmann, W. Combined interventional stroke therapy using intracranial stent and local intra-arterial thrombolysis (LIT). *Neuroradiology*, 2010, 53, 273–282.

[30] Costalat, V; Machi, P; Lobotesis, K; Maldonado, I; Vendrell, JF; Riquelme, C; Mourand, I; Milhaud, D; Héroum, C; Perrigault, PF; Arquizan, C; Bonafé, A. Rescue, combined, and stand-alone thrombectomy in the management of large vessel occlusion stroke using the solitaire device: a prospective 50-patient single-center study: timing, safety, and efficacy. *Stroke*, 2011, 42, 1929-1935.

[31] Nogueira, RG; Levy, EI; Gounis, M; Siddiqui, AH. The Trevo device: preclinical data of a novel stroke thrombectomy device in two different animal models of arterial thrombo-occlusive disease. *J NeuroIntervent* Surg, 2011 Aug 20. [Epub ahead of print]

[32] Mendonça, N; Flores, A; Pagola, J; Rubiera, M; Rodríguez-Luna, D; De Miquel, MA; Cardona, P; Quesada, H; Mora, P; Alvarez-Sabín, J; Molina, C; Ribó, M. Trevo System: Single-Center Experience with a Novel Mechanical Thrombectomy Device. *J Neuroimaging*, 2011 Dec 30. [Epub ahead of print]

[33] Mourand, I; Brunel, H; Costalat, V; Riquelme, C; Lobotesis, K; Milhaud, D; Héroum, C; Arquizan, C; Moynier, M; Bonafé, A. Mechanical Thrombectomy in Acute Ischemic Stroke: Catch Device. *Am J Neuroradiol*, 2011, 32, 1381-1385.

[34] Baker, WL; Colby, JA; Tongbram, V; Talati, R; Silverman, IE; White, CM; Kluger, J; Coleman, CI. Neurothrombectomy devices for the treatment of acute ischemic stroke: state of the evidence. *Ann Intern Med*, 2011, 154, 243-252.

[35] Meyers, PM; Schumacher, HC; Connolly, ES Jr; Heyer, EJ; Gray, WA; Higashida, RT. Current status of endovascular stroke treatment. *Circulation*, 2011, 123, 2591-2601.

[36] Solitaire FR with the Intention for Thrombectomy (SWIFT). http://clinicaltrials.gov/ct2/show/NCT01054560.

[37] Thrombectomy Revascularization of Large Vessel Occlusion in Acute Ischemic Stroke (TREVO). http://clinicaltrials.gov/ct2/show/NCT01088672.

[38] Khatri, P; Hill, MD; Palesch, YY; Spilker, J; Jauch, EC; Carrozzella, JA; Demchuk, AM; Martin, R; Mauldin, P; Dillon, C; Ryckborst, KJ; Janis, S; Tomsick, TA; Broderick, JP; Interventional Management of Stroke III Investigators. Methodology of the Interventional Management of Stroke III Trial. *Int J Stroke*, 2008, 3, 130-137.

[39] Mechanical Retrieval and Recanalization of Stroke Clots Using Embolectomy (MR-RESCUE). http://clinicaltrials.gov/ct2/show/NCT00389467.

[40] DWI/PWI and CTP assessment in the triage of wake-up and late presenting strokes undergoing neurointervention (DAWN). http://www.strokecenter.org/trials/clinicalstudies/dwipwi-and-ctp-assessment-in-the-triage-of-wake-up-and-late-presenting-strokes-undergoing-neurointervention.

[41] Phatouros, CC; Higashida, RT; Malek, AM; Smith, WS; Mully, TW; DeArmond, SJ; Dowd, CF; Halbach, VV. Endovascular stenting of an acutely thrombosed basilar artery: technical case report and review of the literature. *Neurosurgery*, 1999, 44, 667-673.

[42] Samaniego, EA; Dabusand, G; Linfante, I. Stenting in the treatment of acute ischemic stroke: literature review. *Front Neurol*, 2011, 2, 76.

[43] Fitzsimmons, BF; Becske, T; Nelson, PK. Rapid stent-supported revascularization in acute ischemic stroke. *Am J Neuroradiol*, 2006, 27, 1132-1134.

[44] Levy, EI; Mehta, R; Gupta, R; Hanel, RA; Chamczuk, AJ; Fiorella, D; Woo, HH; Albuquerque, FC; Jovin, TG; Horowitz, MB; Hopkins, LN. Self-expanding stents for recanalization of acute cerebrovascular occlusions. *Am J Neuroradiol*, 2007, 28, 816-22.

[45] Zaidat, OO; Wolfe, T; Hussain, SI; Lynch, JR; Gupta, R; Delap, J; Torbey, MT; Fitzsimmons, BF. Interventional acute ischemic stroke therapy with intracranial self-expanding stent. *Stroke*, 2008, 39, 2392-2395.

[46] Brekenfeld, C; Schroth, G; Mattle, HP; Do, DD; Remonda, L; Mordasini, P; Arnold, M; Nedeltchev, K; Meier, N; Gralla, J. Stent placement in acute cerebral artery occlusion:

use of a self-expandable intracranial stent for acute stroke treatment. *Stroke*, 2009, 40, 847-852.

[47] Mocco, J; Hanel, RA; Sharma, J; Hauck, EF; Snyder, KV; Natarajan, SK; Linfante, I; Siddiqui, AH; Hopkins, LN; Boulos, AS; Levy, EI. Use of a vascular reconstruction device to salvage acute ischemic occlusions refractory to traditional endovascular recanalization methods. *J Neurosurg*, 2010, 112, 557-562.

[48] Suh, SH; Kim, BM; Roh, HG; Lee, KY; Park, SI; Kim, DI; Kim, DJ; Nam, HS; Choi, HS. Self-expanding stent for recanalization of acute embolic or dissecting intracranial artery occlusion. *Am J Neuroradiol*, 2010, 31, 459-463.

[49] Linfante, I; Samaniego, EA; Geisbüsch, P; Dabus, G. Self-expandable stents in the treatment of acute ischemic stroke refractory to current thrombectomy devices. *Stroke*, 2011, 42, 2636-2638.

[50] Nakano, S; Iseda, T; Yoneyama, T; Kawano, H; Wakisaka, S. Direct percutaneous transluminal angioplasty for acute middle cerebral artery trunk occlusion: an alternative option to intra-arterial thrombolysis. *Stroke*, 2002, 33, 2872–2876.

[51] Qureshi, AI; Siddiqui, AM; Suri, MF; Kim, SH; Ali, Z; Yahia, AM; Lopes, DK; Boulos, AS; Ringer, AJ; Saad, M; Guterman, LR; Hopkins, LN. Aggressive mechanical clot disruption and low-dose intra-arterial third-generation thrombolytic agent for ischemic stroke: a prospective study. *Neurosurgery*, 2002, 51, 1319–1329.

[52] Jovin, TG; Gupta, R; Uchino, K; Jungreis, CA; Wechsler, LR; Hammer, MD; Tayal, A; Horowitz, MB. Emergent stenting of extracranial internal karotid artery occlusion in acute stroke has a high revascularization rate. *Stroke*, 2005, 6, 2426–2430.

[53] Levy, EI; Siddiqui, AH; Crumlish, A; Snyder, KV; Hauck, EF; Fiorella, DJ; Hopkins, LN; Mocco, J. First Food and Drug Administration-approved prospective trial of primary intracranial stenting for acute stroke: SARIS (stent-assisted recanalization in acute ischemic stroke). *Stroke*, 2009, 40, 3552-3556.

[54] Levy, EI; Rahman, M; Khalessi, AA; Beyer, PT; Natarajan, SK; Hartney, ML; Fiorella, DJ; Hopkins, LN; Siddiqui, AH; Mocco, J. Midterm clinical and angiographic follow-up for the first Food and Drug Administration-approved prospective, Single-Arm Trial of Primary Stenting for Stroke: SARIS (Stent-Assisted Recanalization for Acute Ischemic Stroke). *Neurosurgery*, 2011, 69, 915-920.

[55] Francis, CW; Blinc, A; Lee, S; Cox, C. Ultrasound accelerates transport of recombinant tissue plasminogen activator into clots. *Ultrasound Med Biol*, 1995, 21, 419–424.

[56] Skoloudík, D; Fadrná, T; Roubec, M; Bar, M; Zapletal, O; Blatný, J; Langová, K; Bardon, P; Sanák, D; Kanovský, P; Herzig, R. Changes in hemocoagulation in acute stroke patients after one-hour sono-thrombolysis using a diagnostic probe. *Ultrasound Med Biol*, 2010, 36, 1052-9.

[57] Skoloudík, D; Fadrná, T; Bar, M; Zapletalová, O; Zapletal, O; Blatný, J; Penka, M; Langová, K; Hlustík, P; Herzig, R; Kanovský, P. Changes in haemocoagulation in healthy volunteers after a 1-hour thrombotripsy using a diagnostic 2-4 MHz transcranial probe. *J Thromb Thrombolysis*, 2008, 26, 119-24

[58] Suchkova, VN; Baggs, RB; Francis, CW. Effect of 40-kHz ultrasound on acute thrombotic ischemia in a rabbit femoral artery thrombosis model: enhancement of thrombolysis and improvement in capillary muscle perfusion. *Circulation*, 2000, 101, 2296-301.

[59] Bardoň, P; Skoloudík, D; Langová, K; Herzig, R, Kaňovský, P. Changes in blood flow velocity in the radial artery during one-hour ultrasound monitoring with a 2-MHz transcranial probe—a pilot study. *J Clin Ultrasound*, 2010, 38, 493-496.
[60] Harvey, EN. Biological aspects of ultrasonic waves, a general survey. *Biol Bull*, 1930, 59, 306-325.
[61] Mahon, BR; Nesbit, GM; Barnwell, SL; Clark, W; Marotta, TR; Weill, A; Teal, PA; Qureshi, AI. North American Clinical Experience with the EKOS MicroLysUS Infusion Catheter for the Treatment of Embolic Stroke. *Am J Neuroradiol*, 2003, 24, 534–538.
[62] IMS II Trial Investigators. The Interventional Management of Stroke (IMS) II Study. *Stroke*, 2007, 38, 2127–2135.
[63] Jonszta, T; Czerný, D; Školoudík, D; Böhm, M; Klement, P; Procházka, V. EkoSonicSVTM Endovascular System for Recanalization of the Basilar Artery Occlusion Report of two cases. *VASA*, 2011, 40, 408-413.
[64] Janjua, N; Alkawi, A; Suri, MF; Qureshi, AI. Impact of arterial reocclusion and distal fragmentation during thrombolysis among patients with acute ischemic stroke. *Am J Neuroradiol*, 2008, 29, 253-258.
[65] Nogueira, RG; Yoo, AJ; Buonanno, FS; Hirsch, JA. Endovascular approaches to acute stroke, Part 2: A comprehensive review of studies and trials. *Am J Neuroradiol*, 2009, 30, 859–875.
[66] Tomsick, T; Broderick, J; Carrozella, J; Khatri, P; Hill, M; Palesch, Y; Khoury, J. Interventional Management of Stroke II Investigators. Revascularization results in the Interventional Management of Stroke II trial. *Am J Neuroradiol*, 2008, 29, 582-587.
[67] Berlis, A; Lutsep, H; Barnwell, S; Norbash, A; Wechsler, L; Jungreis, C; Woolfenden, A; Redekop, G; Hartmann, M; Schumacher, M. Mechanical thrombolysis in acute ischemic stroke with endovascular photoacoustic recanalization. *Stroke*, 2004, 35, 1112-1116.
[68] Rohde, S; Haehnel, S; Herweh, C; Pham, M; Stampfl, S; Ringleb, PA; Bendszus, M. Mechanical thrombectomy in acute embolic stroke: preliminary results with the revive device. *Stroke*, 2011, 42, 2954-2956.
[69] Knauth, M. European Launch Of Penumbra Separator™ 3D. The Working Group In Interventional Neuroradiology (WIN) Seminar, Val D'Isere, France, 15 Jan 2012.
[70] Gonzalez, RG; Hirsch, JA; Lev, MH; Schaeffer, P; Schwam, LH. (Eds) Acute Ischemic Stroke: Imaging and Intervention. 2nd Edition. Berlin Heidelberg, Germany: Springer-Verlag; 2011:273.

In: New Developments in Angiography Research
Editors: K. I. Sanders and A. M. Jackson
ISBN: 978-1-62081-492-5

Chapter II

COMPUTED TOMOGRAPHY ANGIOGRAPHY: CLINICAL APPLICATIONS IN CARDIOVASCULAR DISEASE

Zhonghua Sun*
Discipline of Medical Imaging, Department of Imaging and Applied Physics,
Curtin University, Perth, Australia

ABSTRACT

Cardiovascular disease is the leading cause of morbidity and mortality in industrialized countries. Early detection and diagnosis are essential for improvement of treatment outcomes and patient management.

Medical imaging plays an important role in this respect, and currently computed tomography (CT) angiography has been considered the preferred imaging modality due to the emergence of multislice CT and subsequent rapid technological developments over the past decades.

The most threatening manifestations of cardiovascular disease are carotid artery stenosis, coronary artery disease, aortic dissection, aortic aneurysm, pulmonary embolism and peripheral arterial disease. This book chapter will provide an overview of the applications of CT angiography in the diagnosis of cardiovascular disease, with a focus on the diagnostic performance of CT angiography compared to invasive angiography.

INTRODUCTION

Cardiovascular disease is the leading cause of morbidity and mortality in advanced countries, and its prevalence is increasing among developing countries [1-3]. Statistics from the WHO indicates that deaths due to cardiovascular disease account for 33.7% of all deaths worldwide; cancer represents 29.5%; other chronic diseases, 26.5%; injury 7%; and communicable diseases 4.6% [4].

* Email: z.sun@curtin.edu.au; Tel: +61-8-9266 7509; Fax: +61-8-9266 2377.

Cardiovascular disease costs more than any other disease [1]. The total direct and indirect cost of cardiovascular disease and stroke in the United States for 2010 is estimated to be $503.2 billion. In contrast, in 2008, the estimated cost of all cancer and benign neoplasms was $228 billion. Taking into consideration of the current global focus on healthcare utilization, costs, and quality, monitoring and understanding the magnitude of healthcare delivery and costs, as well as the quality of healthcare delivery in relation to cardiovascular disease, are essential.

The most threatening manifestations of cardiovascular disease are carotid artery stenosis, coronary artery disease, aortic dissection, aortic aneurysm, pulmonary embolism, and peripheral arterial disease with potentially fatal consequences of stroke, myocardial infarction, hypertension, or limb loss [5-7]. Cardiovascular disease is not only life threatening but also presents a major economic burden to the healthcare system. Therefore, early detection and diagnosis or disease screening is of paramount importance for improving the treatment outcome and patient management. In this regard, medical imaging plays an important role in the diagnostic management of patients with suspected cardiovascular disease.

Invasive angiography is a radiographic technique used to diagnose vascular disease of the main aortic artery and its distal branches such as those supplying the lower extremities. It is the method of choice for cardiovascular imaging owing to its high spatial and temporal resolution which is still unsurpassed by other imaging modalities.

However, it is an invasive and expensive procedure with associated morbidity and mortality [8]. Furthermore, invasive angiography usually requires a short hospital stay and causes discomfort for the patients.

Therefore, less invasive techniques for imaging and diagnosing cardiovascular disease are being explored, with rapid developments taking place over the last decades. These techniques include computed tomography (CT), magnetic resonance imaging (MRI), and ultrasound and nuclear medicine [9]. Of these imaging modalities, CT is a fast-growing technique reflected in the emergence and wide availability of multislice CT (MSCT) scanners [10-12].

1. Computed Tomography-Technical Developments

MSCT, also known as multidetector CT or multisection CT, represents a significant breakthrough in CT technology. While dual-slice CT has been available since 1992, the first 4-slice CT scanners were introduced in 1998 [10, 13].

Systems with 16- and 64-slice CT have become widely available over the past years, and scanners with 256- and 320-slice have been recently introduced [14-16]. MSCT has been rapidly accepted in the radiological community, which is reflected in the exploding growth in the number of CT examinations and the use of these scanners in clinical practice.

Over the last decade MSCT has undergone rapid technical developments, and has demonstrated regular technical improvements starting with the early generation of 4-slice to 16-slice, 64-slice and up till the most recent models of 320-slice scanners.

The ability of 4-slice CT with gantry rotation time of 500 ms with temporal resolution of 250 ms to image and diagnose cardiovascular disease less invasively has attracted great attention to clinicians in the medical field, and this is represented by the increasing publications of 4-slice CT angiography in the literature [17-19]. Earlier studies with 4-slice CT showed promising results as a less-invasive technique in cardiovascular imaging, however, its diagnostic value was insufficient to replace invasive angiography due to limited spatial and temporal resolution.

With the introduction of 16-and 64-slice CT, image quality in MSCT has become more consistent with improved results achieved [20-22]. With gantry rotation times down to 330 ms for 64-slice CT, temporal resolution for cardiac CT imaging is also markedly improved, and this allows for evaluation of cardiovascular anatomy, including main arteries and associated side branches, even if reliable assessment of the small vessels such as coronary arteries.

In contrast to early generations, 64-slice CT shows improved diagnostic accuracy in cardiovascular disease because of increased spatial and temporal resolution. Isotropic volume data (0.6 x 0.6 x 0.6 mm^3) is possible with 64-slice CT, and the scanning time is reduced to less than 12-15 seconds, allowing a decreased breath-hold time, better utilization of contrast medium with fewer enhancements of adjacent structures and a lower dose of contrast medium.

Improvement of image quality has also been reported in the visualization of cardiovascular system with high sensitivity and specificity achieved [12, 22-24] (Figure 1).

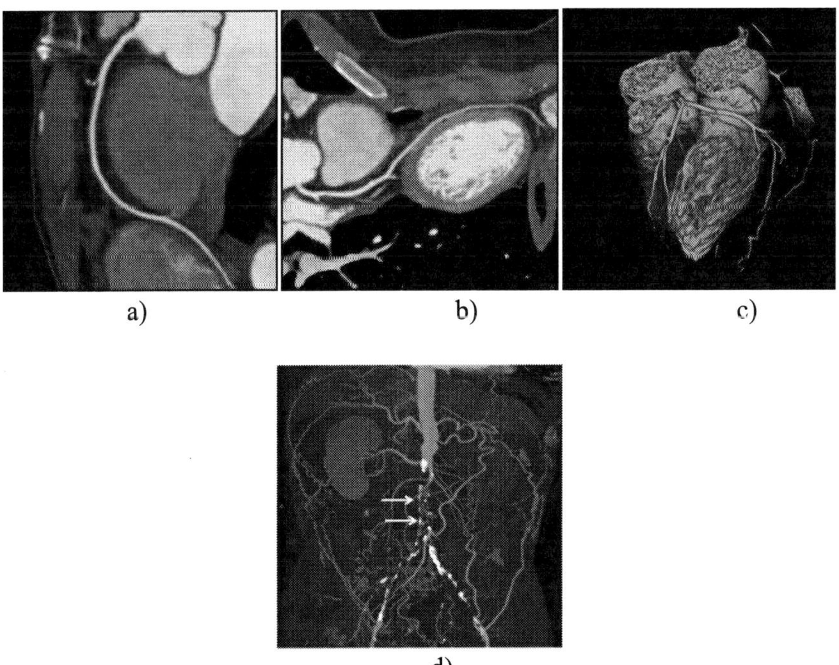

Figure 1. Curved planar reformatted images acquired with 64-slice CT angiography clearly show the right coronary artery (A) and left anterior descending without presence of motion-related artifacts (B). 3D volume rendering demonstrates excellent visualization of the coronary artery and side branches (C). Coronal maximum-intensity projection (MIP) shows an occluded aortic aneurysm with extensive calcification in the infrarenal aorta, extending to the common iliac arteries (arrows in D).

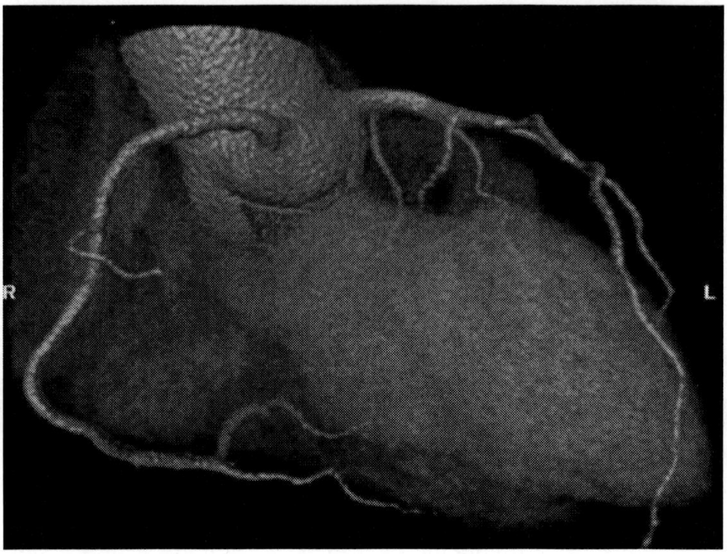

Figure 2. 3D volume rendering of the coronary arteries and side branches are clearly demonstrated with use of 320-slice CT angiography acquired within a single heartbeat with excellent image quality.

Further technical developments in MSCT include introduction of 256- and 320-slice CT scanners into clinical practice. Although no improvements in temporal resolution are observed with these two latest scanners, extended coverage along the longitudinal direction (z-axis) allows for acquisition of volume data in a very short period, and this has been confirmed to be very useful in cardiac imaging [14-16].

For example, with 320-slice CT, a 16 cm of craniocaudal coverage can be obtained in a single heart beat, with excellent image quality and demonstration of the entire coronary arteries, therefore, the entire cardiac volume data can be acquired within one second without requirement of patient movement during the scan (Figure 2).

2. Computed Tomography Angiography

A significant advantage and development of spiral CT data acquisition is its application in 3D imaging of the vascular structures with an intravenous injection of contrast medium. This application is referred to as CT angiography (CTA).

CTA acquires images when blood vessels are fully opacified through intravenous administration of contrast medium to demonstrate either arterial or venous phase enhancement, depending on the scan delay of contrast enhancement. CTA produces angiography-like images non-invasively in a 3D format, thus, it has been increasingly used as a less invasive alternative to invasive angiography in many clinical applications.

Diagnostic value of CT angiography has been significantly advanced with use of MSCT techniques, due to its improved resolution, allowing excellent visualization of both main artery and side branches. CTA has been widely reported to investigate cardiovascular system in terms of both normal anatomy and abnormal changes, and it has been regarded as one of the most valuable applications in CT imaging.

3. Applications of CT Angiography in Cardiovascular Disease

MSCT angiography has proved to be superior to invasive angiography in the diagnosis of many cardiovascular disease, thus, it has been extensively used as the method of choice in the diagnostic applications of cardiovascular imaging.

The following sections present clinical applications of MSCT angiography in a number of common cardiovascular diseases, with a focus on the diagnostic accuracy when compared to invasive angiography.

3.1. Carotid Artery Stenosis

Atherosclerosis is a problem that affects millions of people worldwide, leading to heart attack and strokes. The causative factors that contribute to the formation of atherosclerotic lesions have been studied extensively. Carotid artery atherosclerosis is a major cause of stroke.

About 30% of patients suffering from ischemic stroke are caused by thromboemboli arising from atherosclerotic lesions leading to an abnormal narrowing at the carotid artery bifurcation [25]. Therefore, a leading index for assessing stroke risk for patients with symptoms of minor ischemic stroke is the degree of stenosis of the carotid artery.

Invasive carotid angiography has been considered the gold standard method for evaluating carotid artery stenosis, but its accuracy is restricted to the assessment of lumen changes instead of assessment of plaque morphology [26, 27]. Moreover, it is associated with procedure-related complications such as an increased risk of thromboembolic events [28].

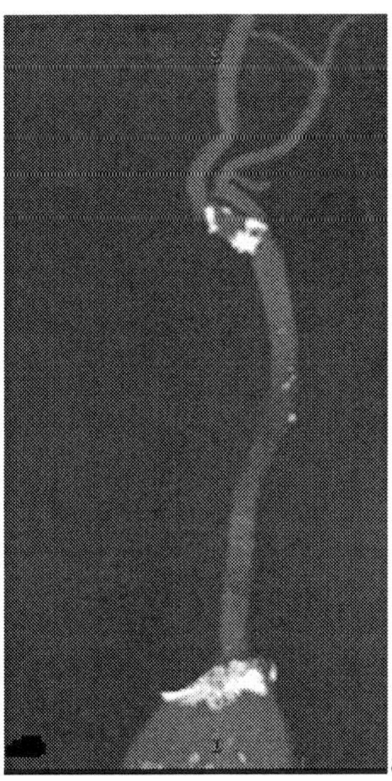
a)

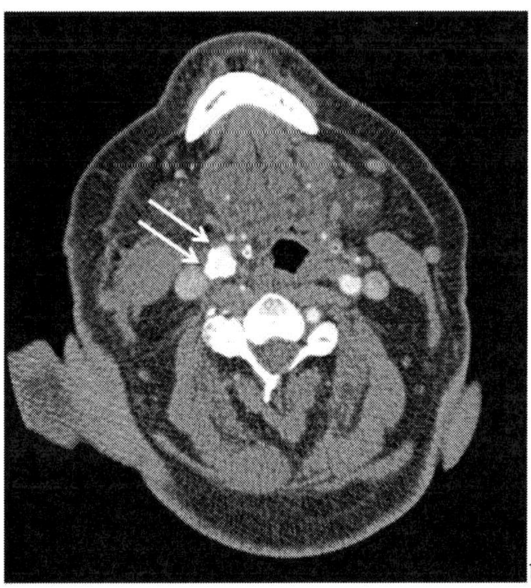
b)

Figure 3. Sagittal MIP shows calcified plaques at the right carotid bifurcation and right internal carotid artery (A). Degree of carotid stenosis cannot be reliably assessed on 2D axial image due to blooming artifact caused by the severe calcification (arrows in B) at the carotid artery.

Consequently, less-invasive imaging techniques such as duplex ultrasound, MSCT angiography and MR angiography have been increasingly studied for diagnosis of carotid artery disease with regard to their potential value when compared to carotid angiography [9, 29]. Despite rapid developments of MSCT imaging over the last decade, CT angiography is not as widely used in imaging and diagnosing carotid artery stenosis as duplex ultrasound and MR angiography. Studies showed that moderate to high diagnostic value was achieved with MSCT angiography for the detection of carotid stenosis [30-32] (Figure 3.A). The main limitation of MSCT angiography is due to the interference of blooming artifacts from severely calcified plaques at the carotid artery, which result in inaccurate assessment of the degree of carotid artery stenosis (Figure 3.B). In contrast, contrast-enhanced MR angiography and duplex ultrasound have been reported to be accurate modalities for the detection of carotid artery stenosis with more than 90% sensitivity achieved using MR angiography and duplex ultrasound when identifying a stenosis of 70% or greater [29, 33, 34]. Moreover, a combination of contrast-enhanced MR angiography and duplex ultrasound was found to increase diagnostic sensitivity close to 100%, indicating the reliability of these non-invasive imaging modalities [32].

3.2. Coronary Artery Disease

Coronary artery disease (CAD) is the leading cause of death in advanced countries. The standard of reference for diagnosis of CAD is still invasive coronary angiography, with the advantage of high spatial resolution and temporal resolution. However, invasive coronary angiography is associated with a small but distinct procedure-related morbidity (1.5%) and mortality (0.2%) rate. Given the invasiveness of coronary angiography and potential danger of having a small risk of serious complications (arrhythmia, stroke, coronary-artery dissection and death), a non-invasive technique for imaging of the coronary artery disease is highly desirable. Over the last decade, great strides have been made in the field of cardiac imaging as non-invasive coronary imaging modalities have undergone rapid developments. Imaging of the heart has moved into a new diagnostic era with the introduction of MSCT and development of electrocardiography-synchronized scanning and reconstruction techniques.

The feasibility of cardiac CT was initially demonstrated with 4-slice CT using retrospective ECG-gated technique. Earlier studies with 4-slice CT showed moderate diagnostic accuracy with pooled sensitivity and specificity of 78%, 93%, respectively [11]. However, image quality was impaired in many cases with 4-slice CT due to limited spatial and temporal resolution, and the unassessable segments could be as high as more than 20% in 4-slice CT studies. With the introduction of 16-slice CT, image quality in MSCT angiography has been improved. Studies that used 16-slice CT with acquisition and rotation times of <400 ms have reported sensitivities between 83% and 98% and specificities between 96% and 98% [11, 35, 36]. Shorter examination times are possible with further improved diagnostic accuracy with 64-slice CT owing to improved spatial and temporal resolution compared with 16-slice CT. Acquisition of isotropic volume data are made available with 64-slice CT, thus, detection of main and side coronary artery branches is improved when compared to earlier types of MSCT scanners. Several meta-analyses of 64-slice CT studies reported that the mean sensitivities of 64-slice CT angiography ranged from 86% to 97% and specificities from 88% to 96% [12, 37, 38].

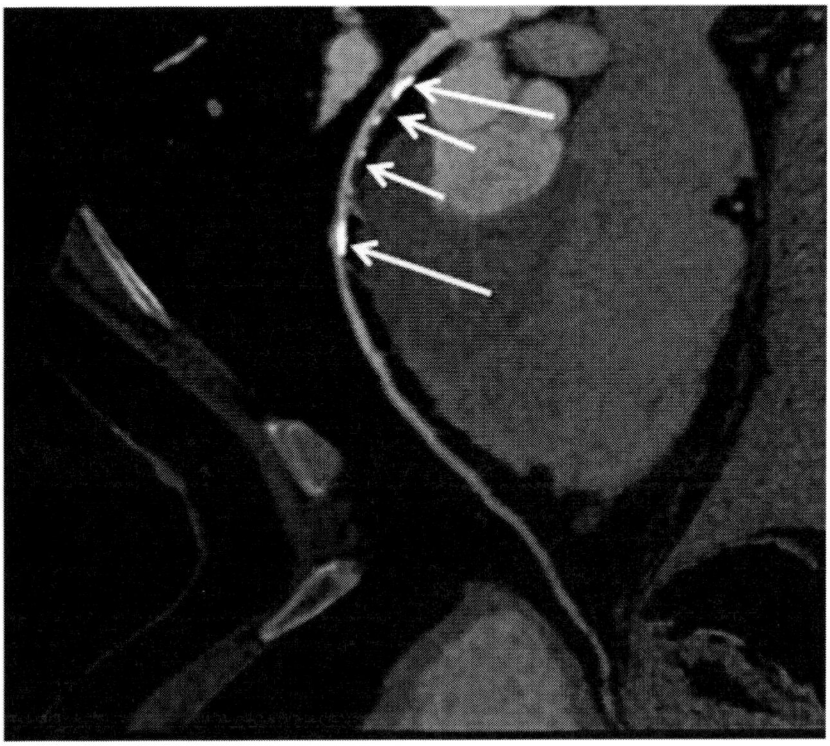

Figure 4. Curved planar reformatted image shows calcified plaques (long arrows) and mixed type of plaques (short arrows) in the proximal segment of right coronary artery.

These studies concluded that MSCT, especially with 64-or more slice CT has high diagnostic accuracy for detection of CAD and could be used as an effective alternative to invasive coronary angiography in selected patients. The introduction of dual-source CT represents another technological improvement of MSCT in cardiac imaging, as the temporal resolution is shortened from 165 ms to 83 ms, and heart rate dependence is eliminated [39]. Studies performed with dual-source CT showed promising results with high diagnostic accuracy for detection of CAD, and most importantly the image quality is independent of heart rate [40-42] (Figure 4). The development of wide-area detector CT enables greater coverage per gantry rotation. Expansion of MSCT systems from a prototype 256-slice to a 320-slice system has allowed for acquisition of whole-heart coverage in one gantry rotation with a slice thickness of 0.5 mm [14-16]. Studies performed with 256- and 320-slice CT demonstrated the ability of CT coronary angiography for quantification of coronary lumen stenosis and assessment of plaque morphology and distribution in the coronary arteries [43-45]. In patients with atrial fibrillation, 320-slice CT was reported to visualize 96% of all coronary segments with sufficient image quality to enable a diagnosis [44, 45].

3.3. Pulmonary Embolism

Pulmonary embolism (PE) is a relatively common vascular disease. Acute PE is the third most common acute cardiovascular disease, after myocardial infarction and stroke [46, 47].

Conventional pulmonary angiography was traditionally regarded as the gold standard for diagnosis of PE. However, it is not only an invasive procedure with risk of mortality (0.5%) and morbidity (6%) [48, 49], but also lacks of diagnostic accuracy as subsegmental clot is not always recognized. Studies have shown that there is considerable interobserver disagreement for the presence or absence of an embolism at pulmonary angiography when looking at small pulmonary arteries, particularly at the subsegmental vessels [50, 51].

With the rapid developments of MSCT techniques, CT pulmonary angiography (CTPA) was initially used as an adjunct and an alternative to other imaging modalities [52], and recently it is widely recognized as the method of choice for diagnosis of suspected PE due to its superior sensitivity and specificity to ventilation-perfusion (V/Q) isotope scanning and other imaging modalities [53-55]. Moreover, CTPA allows a quantitative assessment which correlates well with clinical severity and has good interobserver agreement. Early studies using single slice and 4-slice CTPA reported moderate diagnostic accuracy or limited visualization of subsegmental clots because of limited spatial and temporal resolution [56, 57]. However, CTPA with defined MSCT protocols using 16-and 64-slice CT allows better identification of both central and peripheral thrombus [51, 52, 58]. Improvements in CT technology allow routine visualization of pulmonary arteries to the subsegmental level, with less motion-related artifact and fewer indeterminate results [59] (Figure 5). Prospective Investigation of Pulmonary Embolism Diagnosis (PIOPED II) represents the best study so far published on CTPA [60]. The high specificity and negative predictive value (>95%) of CTPA indicates that the diagnosis of PE can be safely excluded by a negative CTPA [60, 61]. In addition to routine CTPA, ECG-gated CT angiography has been recommended during pulmonary CTA due to the following reasons: first, right ventricular function can be assessed with the aim of stratifying patients with right ventricular dysfunction, thus, guiding therapeutic decisions; second, ECG-gated CTA serves dual purposes of assessing both coronary artery disease and PE, as clinical signs and symptoms of PE and myocardial infarction overlap [62]. Therefore, this protocol could improve patient evaluation and triage, especially in the emergency department [59]. Although dual-source CT was developed mainly to achieve high temporal resolution for cardiac imaging [39-42], it resolved a major drawback of contrast-enhanced applications with dual-energy differentiation. The application of dual-energy pulmonary CTA in the diagnosis of PE primarily relies on the ability to identify contrast medium or specific tissue infiltration, which cannot be precisely detected with single energy CT [63]. Recent studies using dual-energy CT have shown that it can provide high-quality morphologic analysis and functional information on the pulmonary circulation from the same dataset, comparable to pulmonary MR angiography or V/Q scintigraphy [63, 64]. It also allows comparison of pulmonary CTA images acquired at different energies in the same patient at the same time point after contrast medium injection [63]. A main disadvantage of dual-energy pulmonary CTA is the higher radiation exposure compared with single source CT, thus, justification of use of this technique in younger patients should be considered to minimize the potential risk of radiation –induced malignancy.

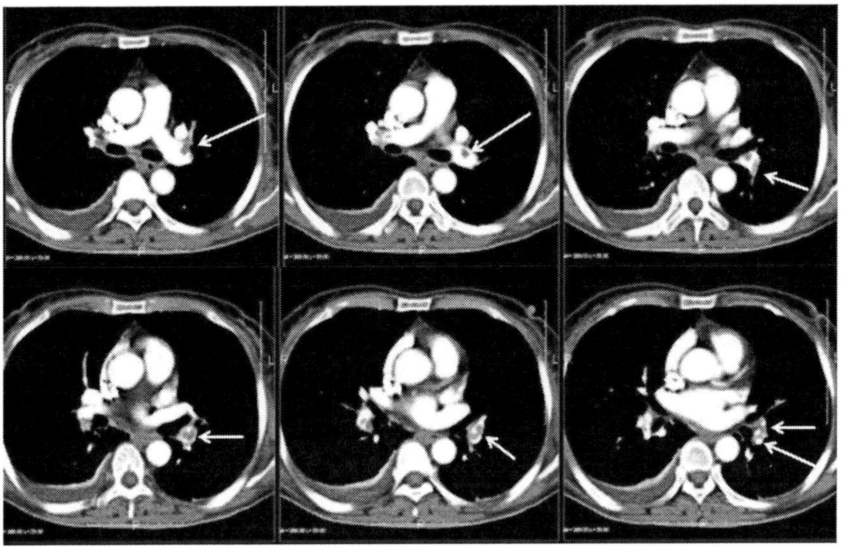

Figure 5. Multiple pulmonary emboli are found in the left main pulmonary artery (long arrows) and left lower lobar and segmental branches (short arrows).

3.4. Aortic Dissection

Aortic dissection is a common vascular disease and it is the most frequent cause of aortic emergency. Aortic dissection can be a life-threatening event which is characterized by splitting of the aortic wall by high blood pressure entering the media through an intimomedial entrance tear. Multislice CT angiography is the preferred method for diagnosis of aortic dissection with a sensitivity and specificity of nearly 100% [65, 66]. CT angiography has been shown to be more sensitive than invasive angiography and is comparable to MR imaging and transesophageal echocardiography for diagnosis of aortic dissection [67, 68]. CT angiography or echocardiography is usually performed in patients in whom acute aortic dissection is clinically suspected on the basis of presentation and initial investigations [69, 70]. A systematic review of the diagnostic accuracy of transoesophageal echocardiography, CT angiography, and MR imaging reported a mean sensitivity and specificity of more than 95% for all three investigations [71]. In addition to assisting the diagnosis of aortic dissection, imaging techniques can help to plan management. Differentiation between true and false lumens is important in the planning of percutaneous treatment with endovascular stent grafts or surgical repair of aortic dissections [72, 73]. It is crucial to identify the lumen of origin in major branch vessels such as coronary, carotid, renal and mesenteric arteries before treatment because viscera supplied by the false lumen are at risk when the false lumen is spontaneously or surgically occluded [74]. Axial CT imaging supplemented by 2D or 3D reconstructions is able to accurately identify the intimal flap which separates the true lumen from the false lumen and determine the type and extent of dissection (Figure 6). 64- and more slice CT with ECG gated CT angiography has allowed the simultaneous imaging of the aorta and coronary and pulmonary arteries, with the potential to accurately diagnose coronary artery disease, pulmonary embolism, and aortic dissection in one method [75]. Thus, CT remains the first choice for diagnostic testing in most centres.

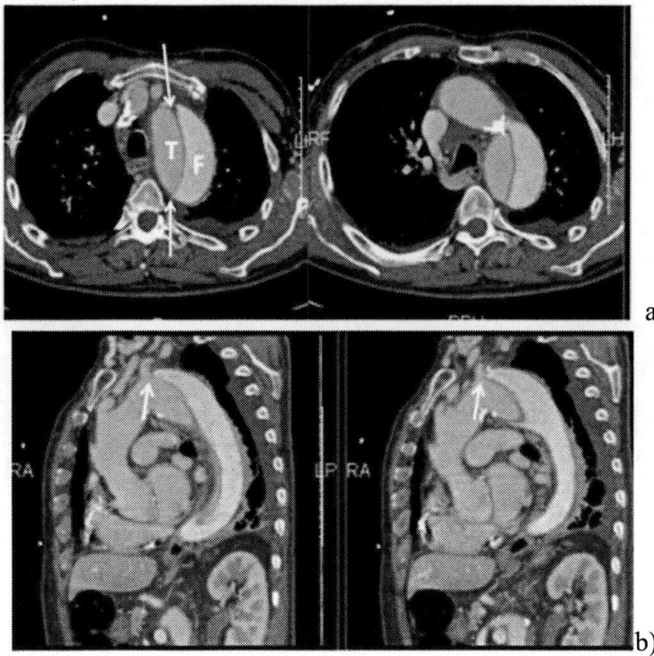

Figure 6. 2D axial image shows Stanford type B dissection involving the aortic arch (A), with intimal tear arising distal to the left subclavian artery (arrows in B) as shown on sagittal reformatted images. Arrows in A indicate the intimal flap. T-true lumen, F-false lumen.

Serial follow-up imaging is important in patients with aortic dissection, and MRI has the advantage in this aspect as it does not involve ionising radiation. Guidelines recommend the use of echocardiography or CT, or both, in the initial imaging of patients suspected of acute aortic dissection, whereas MRI is favoured for the assessment of chronic dissection [76]. Invasive angiography is only reserved in patients in whom visceral malperfusion is suspected or percutaneous treatment with endovascular stent grafts is being considered.

3.5. Abdominal Aortic Aneurysm

Abdominal aortic aneurysm (AAA) is a common vascular disease that affects the elderly population. Most of the AAAs (>80%) are located in an infrarenal position, while only a small percentage of them belong to juxtarenal or suprarenal AAAs. Common risk factors attributable to the development of AAA include increased age, smoking, atherosclerosis and hypertension [77]. AAAs are about three to four times more common in men than in women. Once an aneurysm has been detected by routine physical exam and radiographic studies, the risk of rupture is weighed against the risk of surgical repair for each individual patient. The major determinant for risk of rupture is aneurysm diameter. Therefore, accurate assessment of the aneurysm size and extent by imaging modalities plays an important role in preoperative planning and postoperative follow-up. While invasive angiography has been losing its dominant role for arterial imaging, spiral CT angiography has been confirmed as the best single imaging technique for both preoperative patient assessment and postoperative surveillance [78, 79].

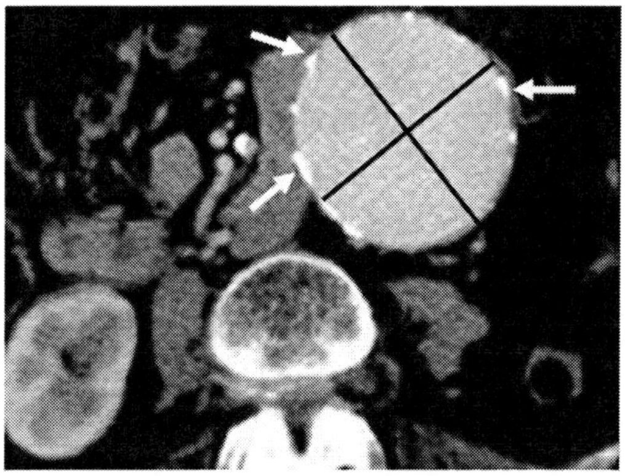

Figure 7. An axial CT image shows a large aortic aneurysm with extensive artery wall calcification. The black lines refer to measurements of the aneurysm diameter at maximal dimensions, while arrows indicate the calcification in the aortic wall.

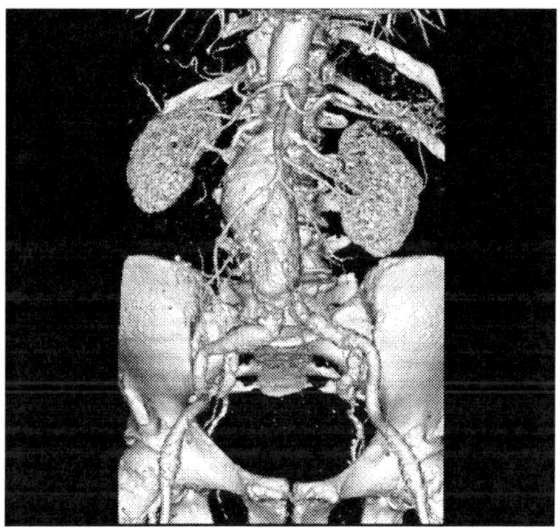

(a)

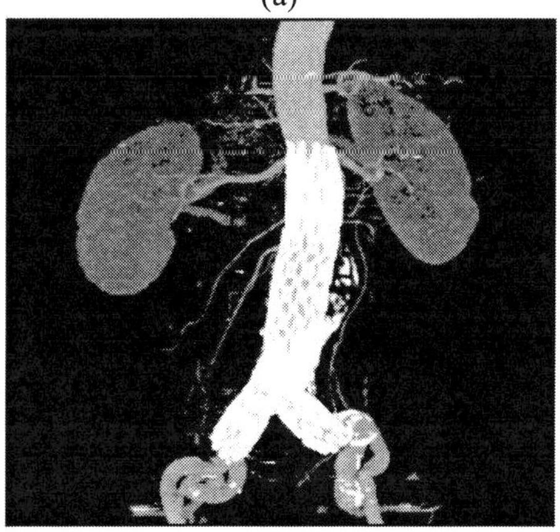

(b)

Figure 8. 3D surface shaded display shows an infrarenal aortic aneurysm involving bilateral common iliac arteries (A). Coronal MIP is a follow-up of a patient treated with suprarenal stent graft with renal arteries patent (B).

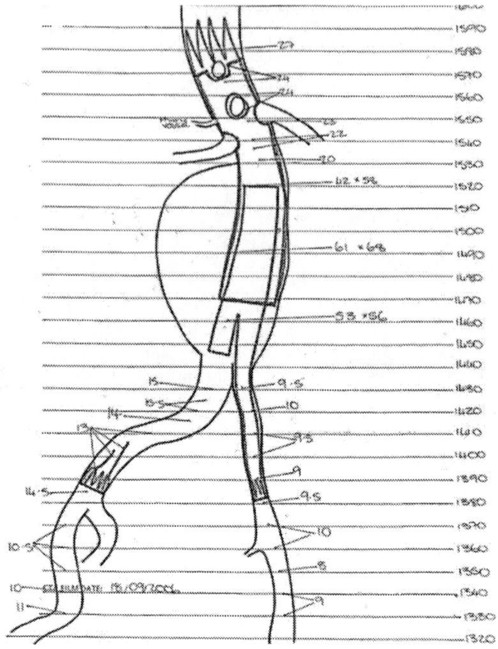

(9a)

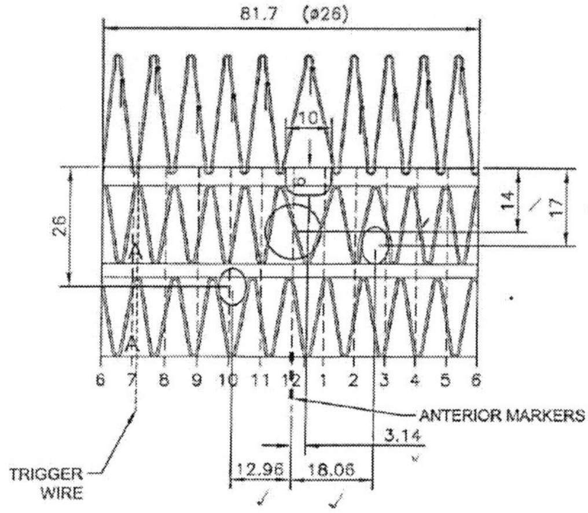

(b)

Figure 9. Diagram shows preoperative planning of endovascular aneurysm repair with detailed measurements of the relevant parameters and design of the stent-graft to be implanted in a patient with aortic aneurysm (A). Viewing from the top to the bottom, scallop fenestration, large fenestration and small fenestrations are recommended for the celiac axis, superior mesenteric artery and bilateral renal arteries, respectively (B).

Axial CT images are most commonly used to determine the maximal aneurysm diameter, including both patent lumen and thrombus (Figure 7). In addition to 2D axial views, a number of postprocessing visualizations such as multiplanar reformation, maximum-intensity projection and volume rendering visualizations are also widely used to enhance the role of CT angiography in preoperative planning. These visualizations provide additional information for assessment of aneurysm extent, and relationship between aneurysms and the arterial branches (Figure 8).

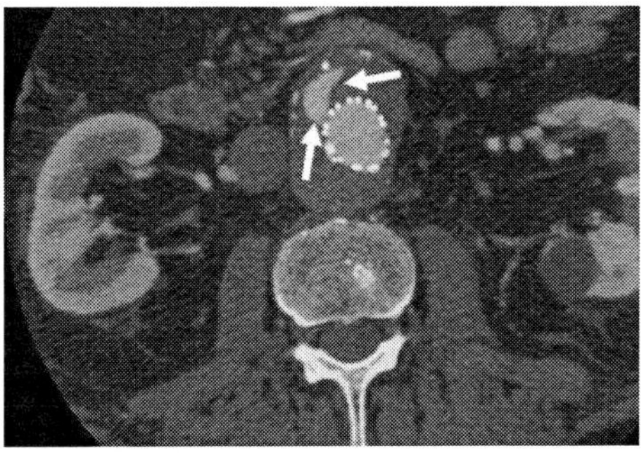

Figure 10. Contrast enhancement is noticed inside the aneurysm sac but outside the stent graft indicating a type I endoleak in the proximal segment of aortic stent graft, as demonstrated on the 2D axial CT image (arrows).

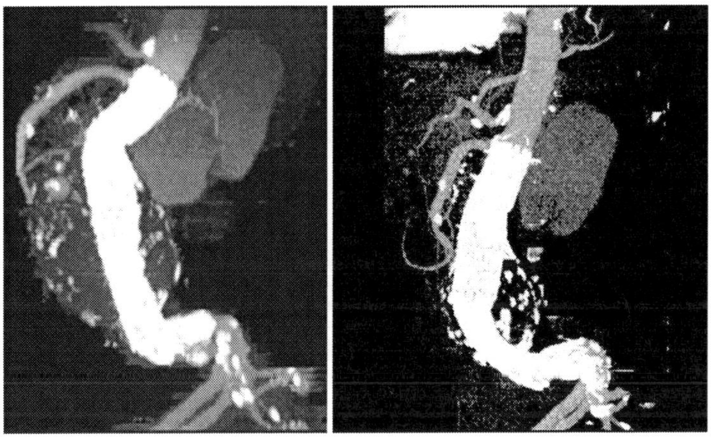

(a) (b)

Figure 11. (A) A stent graft migration of 10.2 mm was observed in a patients treated with suprarenal stent graft due to foreshortening of the longitudinal aneurysm sac at the 24-month follow up (B).

Preoperative measurements include the diameter and length of the aneurysm, the aneurysm's centre line with respect to any curvature of the aorta, the diameter of the aneurysm neck, the neck length (distance from the lowest level of the renal arteries to the proximal segment of the aneurysm), and the diameter and length of the common iliac arteries (Figure 9) [80, 81]. As a less invasive technique, endovascular aneurysm repair (EVAR) was introduced two decades ago for repair of aortic aneurysms, and technical developments allowed it to be used as an effective alternative to open surgical repair, especially in patients with comorbid conditions. Randomized controlled trials have reported that EVAR has lower 30-day mortality than the open surgery repair of AAA [82, 83]. Subsequent reports on the endovascular repair of AAA, which is based on mid-term to long-term follow-up, confirmed that the technique is safe and has no significant effect on renal function [84-87]. CT angiography has been routinely used to monitor the success of EVAR [79-81, 88-90]. CT angiography involves a series of diameter measurements of the aneurysm at regular intervals to determine whether the aneurysm is shrinking, enlarging or unchanged, or detection of procedure-related complications such as endoleaks (Figure 10) or stent graft migration (Figure 11).

3.6. Peripheral Arterial Disease

Peripheral arterial disease (PAD) is an important health problem with a high prevalence in the industrialized countries [91]. It is associated with a clinical situation resulting from altered tissue perfusion, which may lead to acute or chronic ischemia. The disease is known to be related to ageing, and unhealthy lifestyles typical of wealthier populations (smoking, high-calorie diet, sedentary lifestyle, etc.). In 95% of cases, it is caused by atherosclerosis and manifests as a diffuse disease with constant involvement of other regions, such as the coronary and carotid arteries [92, 93]. For many years, invasive angiography with arterial catheterization was the main diagnostic technique for surgical planning and endovascular treatment of PAD. However, it is an invasive technique that requires hospitalization and is burdened by a small risk of immediate (dissection, mobilization of atheromatous plaques or microemboli) and late (pseudoaneurysms) complications [94, 95]. Diagnostic value of invasive angiography in many vascular regions has been challenged over the last decade with the rapid development of non-invasive imaging methods like CT angiography, MR angiography and colour Doppler ultrasound. CT angiography performed with multislice scanners and a large number of detectors is a rapid, less invasive and well-established technique that enables scanning of long segments of the vascular tree during a single breathhold with thinner section thickness [96, 97]. Combined sensitivity, specificity and accuracy of MSCT angiography were reported to be more than 90% at overall assessment and at aortoiliac and femoro-popliteal levels [98-101], while in the level of infrapopliteal, the diagnostic value of CT angiography with 4-slice CT scanners decreased significantly due to limited spatial resolution [102]. This limitation was resolved with the development of 16-slice and 64-slice CT scanners.

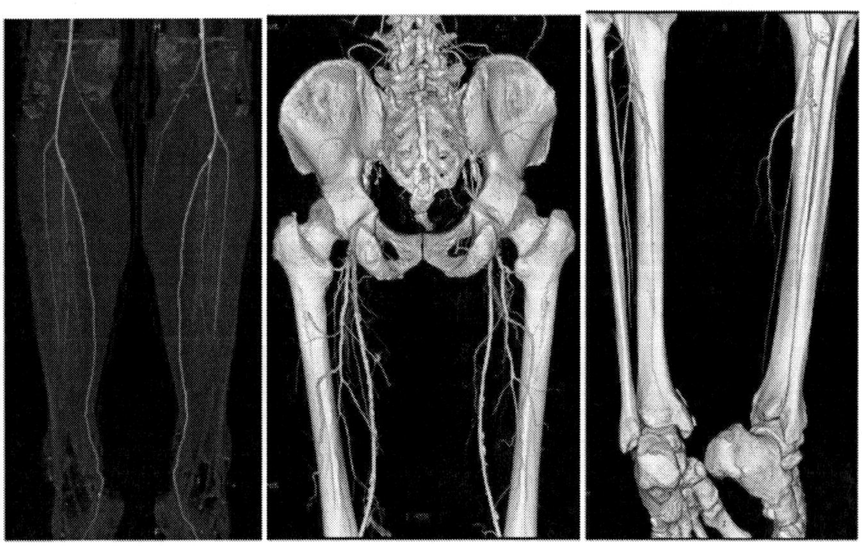

(a) (b) (c)

Figure 12. Coronary MIP image acquired with 64-slice CT angiography clearly demonstrates the femoral and tibial arteries as well as small arterial branches in the lower extremity (A). 3D volume rendering images in another patient show atherosclerotic plaques in the aortoiliac-femoral axis and leg vessels (B, C).

A systematic review reported that diagnostic accuracy of MSCT angiography has been significantly improved with 16-slice CT scanners compared to 4-slice CT scanners, with high sensitivity, specificity and accuracy (more than 96%) achieved in all three anatomic levels (aortoiliac, femoro-popliteal and infrapopliteal) [103]. A recent study with use of 64-slice CT reported very high diagnostic value of CT angiography in detecting significant lesions in peripheral arterial occlusive disease compared to 4- and 16-slice CT [104]. The high spatial and temporal resolution of 64-slice CT enables excellent visualization of aortoiliac and distal arterial branches, thus, overcoming limitations of earlier generations of CT scanners (Figure 12). MSCT angiography was also found to be superior to invasive angiography in visualization of more vascular segments, especially within calf vessels [103].

Invasive angiography was performed in a manner that likely results in an underestimation of patent calf vessels. More patent calf vessels could be visualized if dedicated calf angiography is performed. However, this involves performing additional runs of angiography examinations with aim to limit contrast dose. With the latest CT scanners, MSCT angiography could be used as a reliable alternative to invasive angiography in the diagnosis of peripheral arterial disease.

4. Challenges and Limitations

Improvement of spatial resolution in CT is of particular importance for the evaluation of cardiovascular system and generation of high quality CT angiographic images. Many cardiovascular structures, especially the coronary arteries, represent small and complex 3D structures that require very high and submillimeter isotropic spatial resolution with longitudinal resolution close or equal to in-plane resolution (0.4-0.6 mm). Isotropic volume data (isotropic voxel 0.5 x 0.5 x 0.5 mm^3 or 0.6 x 0.6 x 0.6 mm^3) is available with 64- or more slice MSCT scanners, which enables excellent visualization of both main and side branches including the tiny coronary artery tree. However, the temporal resolution of current MSCT scanners (75 ms) is still inferior to that of invasive coronary angiography (20 ms), thus, further technical improvement is needed to improve image quality of MSCT angiography in patients with high heart rates.

It has been well established that the diagnostic value of CT angiography is hindered by the presence of extensive calcification in the tree wall, and this is especially obvious in the assessment of carotid and coronary artery disease. According to several meta-analyses [12, 37, 38], high-density calcification produces blooming artifacts which lead to overestimation of the degree of coronary stenosis, thus resulting in low positive predictive value (Figure 13). Results from some prospective studies showed that a high patient-based specificity of more than 90% was achieved when patients with body mass index (BMI) >40 kg/m^2 and a calcium score of more than 600 were excluded from the analysis, whereas a low to moderate specificity of 64% and 83% was reported in the studies with inclusion of patients with poor image quality and extensive calcification [105-107]. These conflicting findings indicate the challenge of CT angiography in patients with suspected CAD in the presence of high calcium scores or extensive calcification, or large BMI.

Radiation exposure associated with CT angiography has increased substantially over the past two decades and it has raised a major concern in the medical field that needs to draw attention of both clinicians and manufacturers.

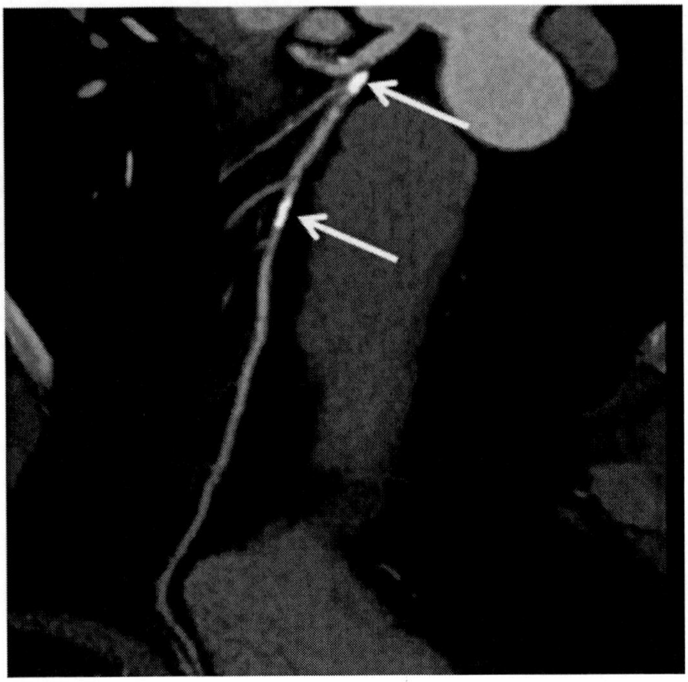

Figure 13. Severely calcified plaques (arrows) in the proximal segment of left anterior descending coronary artery lead to overestimation of the degree of lumen stenosis due to blooming artifacts.

The general view about radiation dose is that CT angiography is associated with a risk of cancer development. The recent Biological Effects of Ionizing Radiation (BEIR) VII provides a framework for estimating cancer risk associated with radiation exposure from ionizing radiation [108]. According to the report, it is estimated that 1 in 1000 people will develop cancer due to an exposure of 10 mSv. Brenner and Hall [109] estimated that approximately 1.5% to 2% of all cancers in the United States may be caused by radiation exposure from CT examinations. Davies *et al.* estimated that in the UK radiation from CT scans causes 800 cancers a year in women and 1300 in men [110]. Radiation exposure is especially important for young and female patients as radiation effects in young patients and women are more severe than in older individuals and in men, so that protection from overly high radiation doses are most important in young individuals. A recent study reported that one in 270 women aged 40 years who undergo coronary CT angiography will develop cancer [111]. Therefore, CT angiography should be performed with dose-saving strategies whenever possible to reduce the radiation dose to patients.

Conclusion

CT angiography has become an important non-invasive imaging modality in the diagnosis of cardiovascular disease. The technological advances in multislice CT gradually overcome the above-mentioned technical and diagnostic challenges, thus, these advances have a dramatic impact on its accuracy to diagnose cardiovascular disease. CT angiography is regarded as the most valuable and effective non-invasive alternative to invasive angiography for the detection and diagnosis of cardiovascular disease. The high diagnostic accuracy of CT angiography has made it a reliable modality in the diagnosis of abdominal aortic aneurysm, aortic dissection, pulmonary embolism and peripheral arterial disease. Although invasive coronary angiography still remains as the gold standard for the diagnosis of coronary artery disease, CT angiography, with the use of 64- or more slice scanners, is a reliable alternative in selected patients. The role of CT angiography will continue to grow with wide availability of multislice CT scanner and its improved capabilities.

References

[1] Lloyd-Jones D, Adams RJ, Brown TM, et al. American Heart Association Statistics Committee and Stroke Statistics Subcommittee. Executive summary: heart disease and stoke statistics 2010 update: A report from the American Heart Association. *Circulation* 2010; 121: 948-954.

[2] Gaziano TA, Bitton A, Anand S, Abrahams-Gessel S, Murphy A. Growing epidemic of coronary heart disease in low-and middle-income countries. *Curr. Probl. Cardiol.* 2010; 35: 72-115.

[3] Liu L. Cardiovascular diseases in China. *Biochem. Cell Biol.* 2007; 85: 157-163.

[4] http://www.who.int/whostat2007/en/index.html

[5] Adams MR, Celermajer DS. Detection of presymptomatic atherosclerosis: a current perspective. *Clin. Sci.* (Lond) 1999; 97: 615-624.

[6] Dormandy J, Heeck L, Vig S. The natural history of claudication: risk to life and limb. *Semin. Vasc. Surg.* 1999; 12: 123-137.

[7] Goyen M, Herborn CU, Kroger K, Lauenstein TC, Debatin JF, Ruehm SG. Detection of atherosclerosis: systemic imaging for systemic disease with whole-body three-dimensional MR angiography-initial experience. *Radiology* 2003; 227: 277-282.

[8] Noto TJ Jr, Johnson LW, Krone R, et al. Cardiac catheterization 1990: a report of the registry of the Society for Cardiac Angiography and Interventions. (SCAandI). *Cathet Cardiovasc. Diagn.* 1991; 24:75–83.

[9] Sun Z, Cao Y, Li H. Multislice computed tomography angiography in the diagnosis of coronary artery disease. *J. Geriatr. Cardiol.* 2011; 104-113.

[10] McCollough CH, Zink FE. Performance evaluation of a multi-slice CT system. *Med. Phys.* 1999;26:2223–30.

[11] Sun Z, Jiang W. Diagnostic value of multislice CT angiography in coronary artery disease: A meta-analysis. *Eur. J. Radiol.* 2006; 60: 279-286.

[12] Sun Z, Lin CH, Davidson R, Dong C, Liao Y. Diagnostic value of 64-slice CT angiography in coronary artery disease: A systematic review. *Eur. J. Radiol.* 2008; 67: 78-84.

[13] Klingenbeck-Regn K, Schaller S, Flohr T et al. Subsecond multi-slice computed tomography: basics and applications. *Eur. J. Radiol.* 1999; 31:110-124.

[14] Chao SP, Law WY, Kuo CJ, Hung HF, Cheng JJ, Lo HM, Shyu KG. The diagnostic accuracy of 256-row computed tomographic angiography compared with invasive coronary angiography in patients with suspected coronary artery disease. *Eur. Heart J.* 2010; 31: 1916-1923.

[15] Rybicki F, Otero H, Steigner M, Vorobiof G, Nallamshetty L, Mitsouras D, Ersoy H, Mather RT, Judy PF, Cai T, Coyner K, Schultz K, Whitmore AG, Di Cardi MF. Initial evaluation of coronary images from 320-detector row computed tomography. *Int. J. Cardiovasc. Imaging* 2008; 24: 535-546.

[16] Dewey M, Deissenrieder ZF, Laule M, Dubel JP, Schlattmann P, Knebel F, Rutsch W, Hamm B. Noninvasive coronary angiography by 320-row computed tomography with lower radiation exposure and maintained diagnostic accuracy: comparison of results with cardiac catheterization in a head-to-head pilot investigation. *Circulation* 2009;120: 867-875.

[17] Nieman K, Oudkerk M, Rensing BJ, van Ooijen P, Munne A, van Geuns RK, et al. Coronary angiography with multi-slice computed tomography. *Lancet* 2001;357:599-603.

[18] Achenbach S, Ulzheimer S, Baum U, et al. Noninvasive coronary angiography by retrospectively ECG-gated multislice spiral CT. *Circulation* 2000;102:2823-2828.

[19] Becker CR, Knez A, Leber A, et al. Detection of coronary artery stenoses with multislice helical CT angiography. *J. Comput. Assist. Tomogr.* 2002;26:750-755.

[20] Hoffman U, Moselewski F, Cury RC, et al. Predictive value of 16 slice multidetector spiral computed tomography to detect significant obstructive coronary artery disease in patients at high risk for coronary artery disease. *Circulation* 2004; 110: 2638-2643.

[21] Deetjen A, Mollmann S, Conradi G, et al. Use of automatic exposure control in multislice computed tomography of the coronaries: comparison of 16-slice and 64-slice scanner data with conventional coronary angiography. *Heart* 2007;93:1040-1043.

[22] Raff GL, Gallagher MJ, O'Neill WW, Goldstein JA. Diagnostic accuracy of non-invasive coronary angiography using 64-slice spiral computed tomography. *J. Am. Coll. Cardiol.* 2005, 46: 552-557.

[23] Fine JJ, Hopkins CB, Ruff N, et al. Comparison of accuracy of 64-slice cardiovascular computed tomography with coronary angiography in patients with suspected coronary artery disease. *Am. J. Cardiol.* 2006, 97: 173-174.

[24] Schuijf JD, Pundziute G, Jukema JW, et al. Diagnostic accuracy of 64-slice multislice computed tomography in the non-invasive evaluation of significant coronary artery disease. *Am. J. Cardiol.* 2006; 98: 145-148.

[25] Leys D. Atherosclerosis: A major health burden. *Cerebrovasc. Dis.* 2001; 11: 1-4.

[26] Streifler JY, Eliaziw M, Fox AJ, et al. Angiographic detection of carotid plaque ulceration: comparison with surgical observations in a multicenter study. *Stroke* 1994; 25: 1130–32.

[27] Walker LJ, IsmailA′, McMeekin W, et al. Computed tomography angiography for the evaluation of carotid atherosclerotic plaque: correlation with histopathology of endarterectomy specimens. *Stroke* 2002; 33: 977–81.

[28] Hessel SJ; Adams DF, Abrams HL. Complications of angiography. *Radiology* 1981; 138: 273–81.

[29] Borisch I, Markus H, Bernhard B, et al. Preoperative Evaluation of Carotid Artery Stenosis: Comparison of contrast-enhanced MR angiography and duplex sonography with digital subtraction angiography. *Am. J. Neuroradiol.* 2003:24: 1117-1122.

[30] Chen CJ, Lee TH, Hsu SH, et al. Multi-Slice CT angiography in diagnosing total versus near occlusions of the internal carotid artery comparison with catheter angiography. *Stroke* 2004; 35: 83-85.

[31] Berg M, Zhang Z, Ikonen A, et al. Multi-detector row CT angiography in the assessment of carotid artery disease in symptomatic patients: comparison with rotational angiography and digital subtraction angiography. *Am. J. Neuroradiol.* 2005; 26: 1022-1033.

[32] Al Shuhaimi A, Ababtain K, Sun Z. Diagnostic value of non-invasive imaging techniques in the detection of carotid artery stenosis: A systematic review. *Radiographer* 2009; 56: 14-18.

[33] Back MR, Wilson JS, Rushing G, et al. Magnetic resonance angiography is an accurate imaging adjunct to duplex ultrasound scan in patient selection for carotid endarterectomy. *J. Vasc. Surg.* 2000; 32(3):429-440.

[34] Clevert DA, Johnson T, Michaely H, et al. High-grade stenoses of the internal carotid artery: Comparison of high-resolution contrast enhanced 3D MRA, duplex sonography and power Doppler imaging. *Eur. J. Radiol.* 2006; 60(3):379-386.

[35] Kuettner A, Trabold T, Schroeder S, Feyter A, Beck T, Brueckner A, et al. Noninvasive detection of coronary artery lesions using 16-detector row multislice spiral computed tomography technology: initial clinical results. *J. Am. Coll. Cardiol.* 2004; 44: 1230-7.

[36] Achenbach S, Ropers S, Pohle FK, et al. Detection of coronary artery stenoses using multi-detector CT with 16x0.75 collimation and 375ms rotation. *Eur. Heart J.* 2005; 26: 1978-1986.

[37] Vanhoenacker PK, Heijenbrok-Kal MH, Van Heste R, Decramer I, Van Hoe LR, Wijns W, et al. Diagnostic performance of multidetector CT angiography for assessment of coronary artery disease: meta-analysis. *Radiology* 2007; 244: 419-428.

[38] Abdulla J, Abildstrom Z, Gotzsche O, Christensen E, Kober L, Torp-Pedersen C. 64-multislice detector computed tomography coronary angiography as potential alternative to conventional coronary angiography: a systematic review and meta-analysis. *Eur. Heart J.* 2007; 28: 3042-3050.

[39] Flohr TG, McCollough CH, Bruder H, Petersilka M, Gruber K, Suss C, et al. First performance evaluation of a dual source CT (DSCT) system. *Eur. Radiol.* 2006; 16: 256-268.

[40] Leber AW, Johnson T, Becker A, von Ziegler F, Tittus J, Nikolaou K, et al. Diagnostic accuracy of dual-source multi-slice CT coronary angiography in patients with an intermediate pretest likelihood for coronary artery disease. *Eur. Heart J.* 2007; 28: 2354-2360.

[41] Brodoefel H, Burgstahler C, Tsiflikas I, Reimann A, Schroeder S, Claussen CD, et al. Dual-source CT: Effect of heart rate, heart rate variability, and calcification on image quality and diagnostic accuracy. *Radiology* 2008; 247: 346-355.

[42] Johnson T, Nikolaou K, Busch S, Leber AW, Becker A, Wintersperger BJ, et al. Diagnostic accuracy of dual-source computed tomography in the diagnosis of coronary artery disease. *Invest. Radiol.* 2007; 42: 484-491.

[43] Mizuno N, Funabashi N, Imada M, Tsunoo T, Endo M, Komuro I. Utility of 256-slice cone beam tomography for real four-dimensional volumetric analysis without electrocardiogram gated acquisition. *Int. J. Cardiol.* 2007; 120:262-267.

[44] Hay CSM, Morse RJ, Morgan-Hughes GJ, Gosling O, Shaw SR, Roobottom CA. Prognostic value of coronary multidetector CT angiography in patients with an intermediate probability of significant coronary heart disease. *Br. J. Radiol.* 2010; 83: 327-330.

[45] Pasricha SS, Nandurkar D, Seneviratne SK, Cameron JD, Crossett M, Schneider-Kolsky, et al. Image quality of coronary 320-MDCT in patients with atrial fibrillation: Initial experience. *AJR Am. J. Roentgenol.* 2009; 193: 1514-1521.

[46] Nikolaou K, Thieme S, Sommer W, Johnson T, Reiser MF. Diagnosing pulmonary embolism: new computed tomography applications. *J. Thorac Imaging* 2010; 25:151–160.

[47] Kelly AM, Patel S, Carlos RC, Cronin P, Kazerooni EA. Multidetector row CT pulmonary angiography and indirect venography for the diagnosis of venous thromboembolic disease in intensive care unit patients. *Acad. Radiol.* 2006; 13:486–495.

[48] Stein PD, Athanasoulis C, Alavi A, Greenspan RH, Hales CA, Saltzman HA, et al. Complications and validity of pulmonary angiography in acute pulmonary embolism. *Circulation* 1992; 85: 462-468.

[49] Mills SR, Jackson DC, Older RA, Heaston DK, Moore AV. The incidence, etiologies, and avoidance of complications of pulmonary angiography in a large series. *Radiology* 1980; 136: 295-299.

[50] Diffin DC, Leyendecker JR, Johnson SP, Zucker RJ, Grebe PJ. Effect of anatomic distribution of pulmonary emboli on interobserver agreement in the interpretation of pulmonary angiography. *AJR Am. J. Roentgenol.* 1998; 171: 1085-1090.

[51] Stein PD, Henry JW, Gottschalk A. Reassessment of pulmonary angiography for the diagnosis of pulmonary embolism: relation of interpreter agreement to the order of the involved pulmonary arterial branch. *Radiology* 1999; 210:689–691.

[52] British thoracic society guidelines for the management of suspected acute pulmonary embolism: British thoracic society standards of care committee pulmonary embolism guideline development group. *Thorax* 2003; 58: 470-484.

[53] Hayashino Y, Goto M, Noguchi Y, Fukui T. Ventilation-perfusion scanning and helical CT in suspected pulmonary embolism: meta-analysis of diagnostic performance. *Radiology* 2005; 234: 740-748.

[54] Guilabert JP, Manzur DN, Tarrasa MJ, Llorens ML, Braun P, Arques MP. Can multislice CT alone run out reliably pulmonary embolism? A prospective study. *Eur. J. Radiol.* 2007; 62: 220-226.

[55] Schoepf UJ, Goldhaber SZ, Costello P. Spiral computed tomography for acute pulmonary embolism. *Circulation* 2004; 109: 2160-2167.

[56] Rathbun SW, Raskob GE, Whitsett TL. Sensitivity and specificity of helical computed tomography in the diagnosis of pulmonary embolism: a systematic review. *Ann. Intern Med.* 2000; 132: 227-232.
[57] van Strijen MJL, de Monye W, Kieft GJ, Pattynama PMT, Prins MH, Huisman MV. Accuracy of single-detector spiral CT in the diagnosis of pulmonary embolism: a prospective multicentre cohort study of consecutive patients with abnormal perfusion scintigraphy. *J. Thromb Haemost.* 2005; 3: 17-25.
[58] Perrier A, Roy PM, Sanchez O, Le Gal G, Meyer G, Gourdier AL, et al. Multidetector-row computed tomography in suspected pulmonary embolism. *N. Engl. J. Med.* 2005; 352: 1760-1768.
[59] Remy-Jardin M, Pistolesi M, Goodman LR, et al. Management of suspected acute pulmonary embolism in the era of CT angiography: a statement from the Fleischner Society. *Radiology* 2007; 245:315–329.
[60] Stein PD, Woodard PK, Weg JG, et al. Diagnostic pathways in acute pulmonary embolism: recommendations of the PIOPED II investigators. *Radiology* 2007; 242:15–21.
[61] Stein PD, Sostman HD, Bounameaux H, et al. Challenges in the diagnosis of acute pulmonary embolism. *Am. J. Med.* 2008; 121:565–571.
[62] Sadigh G, Kelly AM, Cronin P. Challenges, controversies and hot topics in pulmonary embolism imaging. *AJR Am. J. Roentgenol.* 2011; 196: 497-515.
[63] Remy-Jardin M, Faivre JB, Pontana F, et al. Thoracic applications of dual energy. *Radiol. Clin. North Am.* 2010; 48:193–205.
[64] Zhang LJ, Zhao YE, Wu SY, Yeh BM, Zhou CS, et al. Pulmonary embolism detection with dual-energy CT: experimental study of dual-source CT in rabbits. *Radiology* 2009; 252: 61-70.
[65] Castaner E, Andreu M, Gallardo X, et al. CT in nontraumatic acute thoracic aortic disease: typical and atypical features and complications. *Radiographics* 2003; 23:S93–110.
[66] Sebastia` C, Pallisa E, Quiroga S, et al. Aortic dissection: diagnosis and follow-up with helical CT. *Radiographics* 1999; 19:45–60.
[67] Cigarroa JE, Isselbacher EM, DeSanctis RW, Eagle KA. Diagnostic imaging in the evaluation of suspected aortic dissection: old standards and new directions. *N. Engl. J. Med.* 1993; 328:35–43.
[68] Small JH, Dixon AK, Coulden RA, Flower CD, Housden BA. Fast CT for aortic dissection. *Br. J. Radiol.* 1996;69:900–905.
[69] Rampoldi V, Trimarchi S, Eagle KA, et al. International Registry of Acute Aortic Dissection (IRAD) Investigators. Simple risk models to predict surgical mortality in acute type A aortic dissection: the International Registry of Acute Aortic Dissection score. *Ann. Thorac. Surg.* 2007; 83: 55–61.
[70] Nienaber CA, Fattori R, Mehta RH, et al. International Registry of Acute Aortic Dissection. Gender-related diff erences in acute aortic dissection. *Circulation* 2004; 109: 3014–21.
[71] Shiga T, Wajima Z, Apfel CC, Inoue T, Ohe Y. Diagnostic accuracy of transesophageal echocardiography, helical computed tomography, and magnetic resonance imaging for suspected thoracic aortic dissection: systematic review and meta-analysis. *Arch. Intern Med.* 2006; 166: 1350–56.

[72] LePage M, Quint LE, Sonnad SS, Deeb GM, Williams DM. Aortic dissection: CT features that distinguish true from false lumen. *AJR Am. J. Roentgenol.* 2001;177: 207–211.

[73] Williams DM, Lee DY, Hamilton BH, et al. The dissection aorta: percutaneous treatment of ischemic complications—principles and results. *J. Vasc. Intervent. Radiol.* 1997;8: 605–625.

[74] Kapoor V, Ferris JV, Fuhrman CR. Intimomedial rupture: A new CT finding to distinguish true from false lumen in aortic dissection. *AJR Am. J. Roentgenol.* 2004; 183: 109-112.

[75] Johnson TR, Nikolaou K, Wintersperger BJ, et al. ECG-gated 64-MDCT angiography in the differential diagnosis of acute chest pain. *JR Am. J. Roentgenol.* 2007; 188: 76–82.

[76] Erbel R, Alfonso F, Boileau C, et al. Task Force on Aortic Dissection, European Society of Cardiology. Diagnosis and management of aortic dissection. *Eur. Heart J.* 2001; 22: 1642–81.

[77] Alcorn HG, Wolfson SK Jr, Sutton-Tyrell K. Risk factors for abdominal aortic aneurysms in older adults enrolled in Cardiovascular Health Study. *Arterioscler. Thromb Vasc. Biol.* 1996; 16:963–970.

[78] Rydberg J, Kopecky KK, Johnson MS, et al. Endovascular repair of abdominal aortic aneurysms: Assessment with multislice CT. *AJR Am. J. Roentgenol.* 2001; 177: 607-614.

[79] Sun Z. Helical CT angiography of abdominal aortic aneurysms treated with suprarenal stent grafting. *Cardiovasc. Intervent. Radiol.* 2003; 26: 290-295.

[80] Rydberg J, Kopecky KK, Lalka SG, et al. Stent grafting of abdominal aortic aneurysms: Pre- and postoperative evaluation with multislice helical CT. *J. Comput. Assit. Tomgr.* 2001; 25(4): 580-586.

[81] Whitaker SC. Imaging of abdominal aortic aneurysm before and after endoluminal stent graft repair. *Eur. J. Radiol.* 2001; 39: 3-15.

[82] Greenhalgh RM, Brown LC, Kwong GP, et al. Comparison of endovascular aneurysm repair with open repair in patients with abdominal aortic aneurysm (EVAR trial1), 30-day operative mortality results: randomised controlled trial. *Lancet* 2004; 364: 843-848.

[83] Prinssen M, Verhoeven EL, Buth J, et al. A randomized trial comparing conventional and endovascular repair of abdominal aortic aneurysms. *N. Engl. J. Med.* 2004; 14 (351): 1607-1618.

[84] O'Donnell M, Sun Z, Winder J, et al. Suprarenal fixation of endovascular aortic stent grafts: Assessment of medium-term to long-term renal function by analysis of juxtarenal stent morphology. *J. Vasc. Surg.* 2007; 45: 694-670.

[85] Lau LL, Hakaim AG, Oldenburg WA, et al. Effect of suprarenal versus infrarenal aortic endograft fixation on renal function and renal artery patency: a comparative study with intermediate follow-up. *J. Vasc. Surg.* 2003;37:1162-8.

[86] Greenberg RK, Chuter TA, Lawrence-Brown M, Haulon S, Nolte L; Zenith Investigators. Analysis of renal function after aneurysm repair with a device using suprarenal fixation (Zenith AAA Endovascular Graft) in contrast to open surgical repair. *J. Vasc. Surg.* 2004;39:1219-28.

[87] Muhs BE, Verhoeven EL, Zeebregts C, et al. Mid-term results of endovascular aneurysm repair with branched and fenestrated endografts. *J. Vasc. Surg.* 2006; 44: 9-15.

[88] Sun Z. Three-Dimensional visualization of suprarenal aortic tent-grafts: Evaluation of migration in midterm follow-up. *J. Endovasc. Ther.* 2006; 1: 85-93.

[89] Sun Z. 3D multislice CT angiography in post-aortic stent grafting: A pictorial essay. *Korean J. Radiol.* 2006; 7: 205-211.

[90] Sun Z, Allen Y, Mwipatayi B, Hartley D, Lawrence-Brown M. Multislice CT angiography of fenestrated endovascular stent grafting of abdominal aortic aneurysms: A pictorial review of 2D/3D visualizations. *Korean J. Radiol.* 2009; 10: 285-293.

[91] Fowkes FG, Housley E, Cawood EH, Macintyre CC, Ruckley CV, Prescott RJ. Edinburgh Artery Study: prevalence of asymptomatic and symptomatic peripheral arterial disease in the general population. *Int. J. Epidemiol.* 1991, 20: 384-392.

[92] Schoen F (1997) Vascular disease. In: Cotran RS, Kumar V, Collins T, Robbins SL (eds) Robbins pathologic basis of disease. Saunders, Philadelphia, pp 537–551.

[93] Cary N (1996) Pathology of peripheral arterial disease. In: Gorodn L (ed) Textbook of vascular medicine. Edward Arnold, London, pp 143–148.

[94] Lilly MP, Reichman W, Sarazen AA Jr et al. Anatomic and clinical factors associated with complications of transfemoral arteriography. *Ann. Vasc. Surg.* 1990; 4:264–269.

[95] Waugh JR, Sacharias N. Arteriographic complications in the DSA era. *Radiology* 1992; 182:243–246.

[96] Fleischmann D, Rubin GD, Paik DS. Stair-step artifacts with single versus multidetector-row helical CT. *Radiology* 2000, 216: 185-196.

[97] Rubin GD, Shiau MC, Leung AN, Kee ST, Logan LJ, Sofilos MC. Aorta and iliac arteries: single versus multiple detector-row helical CT angiography. *Radiology* 2000, 215: 670-676.

[98] Ofer A, Nitechi SS, Linn S, Epelman M, Fischer D, Karram T, Litmanovich D, Schwartz H, Hoffman A, Engel A. Multidetector CT angiography of peripheral vascular disease: A prospective comparison with intraarterial digital subtraction angiography. *Am. J. Roentgenol.* 2003, 180: 719-724.

[99] Willman JK, Baumert B, Schertler T, Wildermuth S, Pfammatter T, Verdun FR, Seifert B, Marincek B, Böhm T. Aortoiliac and lower extremity arteries assessed with 16-detector row CT angiography: prospective comparison with digital subtraction angiography. *Radiology* 2005, 236: 1083-1093.

[100] Portugaller HR, Schoellnast H, Hausegger KA, Tiesenhausen K, Amann W, Berghold A. Multislice CT angiography in peripheral arterial disease: a valuable tool in detecting significant arterial lumen narrowing? *Eur. Radiol.* 2004,14: 1681-1687.

[101] Ota H, Takase K, Igarashi K, Chiba Y, Haga K, Saito H, Takahashi S. MDCT compared with digital subtraction angiography for assessment of lower extremity arterial occlusive disease: importance of reviewing cross-sectional images. *Am. J. Roentgenol.* 2004, 182: 201-209.

[102] Edwards AJ, Wells IP, Roobottom CA. Multidetector row CT angiography of the lower limb arteries: a prospective comparison of volume-rendered techniques and intra-arterial digital subtraction angiography. *Clin. Radiol.* 2005, 60: 85-95.

[103] Sun Z. Diagnostic accuracy of multislice CT angiography in peripheral vascular disease. *J. Vasc. Intervent. Radiol.* 2006; 17: 1915-1921.

[104] Cernic S, Mucelli FP, Pellegrin A, Pizzolato R, Cova MA. Comparison between 64-row CT angiography and digital subtraction angiography in the study of lower extremities: personal experience. *Radiol. Med.* 2009; 114: 11150-1129.

[105] Miller JM, Rochitte CE, Dewey M, et al. Diagnostic performance of coronary angiography by 64-row CT. *N. Engl. J. Med.* 2008; 359: 2324-2336.

[106] Budoff MJ, Dowe D, Jollis JG, et al. Diagnostic performance of 64-multidetector row coronary computed tomographic angiography for evaluation of coronary artery stenosis in individuals without known coronary artery disease: results from the prospective multicenter ACCURACY (Assessment by Coronary Computed Tomographic Angiography of Individuals Undergoing Invasive Coronary Angiography) trial. *J. Am. Coll. Cardiol.* 2008;52:1724-1732.

[107] Meijboom WB, Meijs MFL, Schuijf JD, et al. Diagnostic accuracy of 64-slice computed tomography coronary angiography: a prospective multicenter, multivendor study. *J. Am. Coll. Cardiol.* 2008; 52:2135-2144.

[108] Committee to Assess Health Risks from Exposure to Low Levels of Ionizing Radiation; Nuclear and Radiation Studies Board, Division on Earth and Life Studies, National Research Council of the National Academies. Health Risks From Exposure to Low Levels of Ionizing Radiation: BEIR VII Phase 2. Washington, DC: The National Academies Press; 2006.

[109] Brenner DJ, Hall EJ. Computed tomography—an increasing source of radiation exposure. *N. Engl. J. Med.* 2007; 357(22):2277–2284.

[110] Davies HE, Wathen CG, Gleeson FV. Risks of exposure to radiological imaging and how to minimise them. *BMJ* 2011; 342: 589-593.

[111] Smith-Bindman R, Lipson J, Marcus R, et al. Radiation dose associated with common computed tomography examinations and the associated lifetime attributable risk of cancer. *Arch. Intern. Med.* 2009; 169: 2078-2086.

In: New Developments in Angiography Research
Editors: K. I. Sanders and A. M. Jackson
ISBN: 978-1-62081-492-5

Chapter III

CATHETER-BASED REGISTRATION AND MOTION COMPENSATION FOR 2-D/3-D FUSION DURING ELECTROPHYSIOLOGY PROCEDURES

Rui Liao*
Siemens Corporate Research, Princeton, NJ, US

ABSTRACT

Radio-frequency catheter ablation (RFCA) of the pulmonary veins (PVs) attached to the left atrium (LA) is usually carried out under fluoroscopy guidance. However, X-ray cannot distinguish well soft tissues, and overlay of detailed anatomical structures via 3-D CT volumes onto the fluoroscopy has shown to help visualization and navigation in Electrophysiology procedures (EP). Registration of the CT volume with the online fluoroscopy however is a challenging task for EP applications duc to the lack of discernable features in fluoroscopic EP images. In addition, respiratory motion may impair the utility of static overlay of the volume with fluoroscopy for catheter navigation. In this chapter, we present a catheter-based method for 2-D/3-D registration and motion compensation for utilizing the 3-D data. In particular, we use the coronary sinus (CS) catheter in bi-plane fluoroscopic images and the coronary sinus in the CT volume as a location constraint to accomplish 2-D/3-D registration. After initial registration using the CS catheter, a B-spline based method for tracking the circumferential lasso catheter in monoplane fluoroscopy is implemented to track the motion at the PVs for a motion-compensated dynamic overlay. Since both the CS catheter and the lasso catheter are typically used during EP procedures, the proposed method does not require additional instruments, and achieves motion estimation right at the site of ablation. In addition, the proposed method only requires bi-plane acquisition of fluoroscopic images at the very beginning for registration purpose, and monoplane fluoroscopy is used for online monitoring and motion compensation during the EP procedures, minimizing the X-ray

* Supported by Siemens Corporate Research. Corresponding author: Rui Liao PhD, Siemens Corporate Research, 755 College Road East, Princeton, NJ 08540, US. Telephone: +1-609-734-6500. Fax: +1-609-734-6565. Email: Rui.Liao@siemens.com.

dose needed. The performance of the proposed tracking algorithm was evaluated on 466 monoplane frames with an average error of 0.66 ± 0.37 mms. Quantitative validation based on simulations and visual inspection on real data further demonstrates the feasibility of the proposed workflow in EP procedures.

Keywords: Image-guided Interventions, Electrophysiology, 2-D/3-D Registration, Motion Compensation, 2-D/3-D Fusion, Augmented Reality, X-ray, Angiography and Fluoroscopy

1. INTRODUCTION

Atrial fibrillation (AF) is one of the most common heart rhythm disorders and a leading cause of stroke [1]. Radio-Frequency catheter ablation (RFCA) has become an accepted option for treating AF in today's EP labs, as an alternative to anti-arrhythmic drugs, cardiac surgery, and external defibrillator [2, 3, 4, 5]. In order to guide the process of finding the site of origin where the excess firing of cells occur, 2-D X-ray fluoroscopy has been routinely used to provide real-time monitoring of EP procedures. However, fluoroscopic images do not display the anatomic structures without the contrast agent, which on the other hand needs to be minimized for patients' safety. In order to augment the doctor's view of the heart anatomies and help navigate the ablation catheters to the pulmonary veins, pre-operative high-quality Computed Tomographic (CT) and/or Magnetic Resonance (MR) volume can be overlaid onto the intra-operative fluoroscopic images during EP procedures [6, 7, 8].

Registration between 3-D volumes and 2-D fluoroscopic images for EP is a challenging task due to the fact that there are few discernable features in a typical EP fluoroscopic image. Rhode et. al. proposed to use multimodality fiducial skin markers to register MR volumes with X-ray images [9]. This method however requires specialized markers as well as a specialized workflow to guarantee that the markers are applied at the same position between the pre- and intra-operative data. In this study, we investigate the feasibility of utilizing coronary sinus (CS) and the catheter placed inside the CS as a location constraint to perform 2-D/3-D registration between the X-ray image and the CT volume.

After 2-D/3-D registration between 3-D volumes and 2-D fluoroscopy, static overlay can be generated to facilitate the EP procedure. However, a static overlay does not follow the heart while it beats and moves through the breathing cycle. This effect may impair the utility of fluoroscopic overlays for catheter navigation. By synchronizing the fluoroscopic images with electrocardiogram (ECG), cardiac motion can be eliminated, and respiratory motion can be isolated for the fused visualization. Motion compensated navigation for coronary intervention was suggested in [10]. The proposed method is based on a magnetic tracking system for device localization and hence is expensive due to the requirement on specialized catheters. Image-based device localization for breathing motion compensation during hepatic artery catheterization and liver embolization was shown in [11] and [12] respectively. Only translational motion in the imaging plane was compensated, which hence is not sufficient for breathing motion compensation for EP applications because the left atrium undergoes three dimensional motions during respiration [13]. In [7, 8] image-based motion compensation for EP was suggested for a biplane system, which is less common than a monoplane system due to its much higher cost. In this study, we investigate the feasibility of tracking in the monoplane fluoroscopy the circumferential lasso catheter that is routinely used in EP procedures.

Since both CS catheter and lasso catheter are routinely used during EP procedures, the proposed workflow does not impose any extra operations on physicians during the procedure. In addition, in EP cases very often the inserted devices (i.e. catheters) are the only structure that is clearly shown in the fluoroscopic images, while other anatomical structures are barely visible when contrast agent is not injected. The proposed method therefore has the advantage of no extra contrast agent administration for patients' safety.

2. METHODS

2.1. CS-Based 2-D/3-D Registration

We rely on a semi-automatic yet minimal user-input method for 2-D segmentation of the CS catheter on a fluoroscopic image, which is reliable and robust even when the signal-to-noise ratio of the fluoroscopic image is relatively low. Firstly, CS catheter is enhanced by Hessian-based filtering as described in [14]. The filter identifies the tubular structures using the eigenvalues λ_1 and λ_2 ($|\lambda_1| << |\lambda_2|$) of the Hessian matrix:

$$\mathbf{H}_\sigma = \sigma^2 \begin{bmatrix} \frac{\partial^2 \mathbf{u}_\sigma}{\partial x^2} & \frac{\partial^2 \mathbf{u}_\sigma}{\partial x\, \partial y} \\ \frac{\partial^2 \mathbf{u}_\sigma}{\partial x\, \partial y} & \frac{\partial^2 \mathbf{u}_\sigma}{\partial y^2} \end{bmatrix} \quad (1)$$

here $\mathbf{u}_\sigma$ is the convolution of the fluoroscopic image with a Gaussian kernel of size σ. Ideally σ should be the radius of the catheter and the direction of the derivative would be the same as the direction of the catheter. The vesselness is calculated as:

$$V_\sigma = \begin{cases} 0 & \lambda_2 < 0 \\ e^{R_B^2/2\beta^2}\left(1 - e^{-S^2/2\alpha^2}\right) & \lambda_2 \geq 0 \end{cases} \quad (2)$$

where $R_B = \lambda_1 / \lambda_2$, $S = \sqrt{\lambda_1^2 + \lambda_2^2}$, and α and β controls the sensitivity of the filter. Secondly, the centerlines of the 2-D catheter of the two fluoroscopic images from plane A and plane B, denoted by C_{2dA} and C_{2dB} respectively, are extracted interactively in a manner similar to Intelligent Scissor (IS) [15]. In particular, when user moves the mouse, the shortest path between a seed point (e.g. one end point of the catheter) and the current mouse position is searched on-the-fly by Fast Marching method [16]. The cost of a path L is:

$$C(L)=\sum_{p=1}^{m}1/(0.001+v(p)^4)+\omega S(L) \tag{3}$$

where $v(p)$ is the vesselness at pixel p, m is the number of pixels on the path L, $S(L)$ is the length of the path L, and ω controls the relative weights of these two factors. It can be seen that a path of a stronger vesselness and a shorter total length is preferred over a path of a weaker vesselness and a longer length. Lastly, the extracted 2-D CS catheter is smoothed by fitting an open-end B-Spline curve that has a minimized weighted summation of the total curvature and the distance to the original centerline.

The centerline of the 3-D CS, denoted by C_{3d}, is extracted automatically from the CT volume based on the method described in [17]. This method is adapted for the typical intensity variation of coronary sinus due to the presence of valves at orifices and insufficient distribution of contrast agent, and addresses the problem of high probability of leaking due to the fact that CS is close to the left coronary arteries, left atrium and left ventricle.

In this study, we assume there is only one global rigid-body transformation relating points in the 3-D volume to points on the fluoroscopic images. We hence need to estimate the rigid-body transformation T consisting of 3 translations and 3 rotations:

$$\arg\min_{T} D_{3d}\left(recon(C_{2dA}, C_{2dB}), T(C_{3d})\right) \tag{4}$$

where $T(C_{3d})$ is the 3-D CS after rigid-body transformation T, $recon$ denotes the process that reconstructs a 3-D curve from two corresponding 2-D curves, and $D_{3d}(C_1, C_2)$ is the 3-D distance between two 3-D curves C_1 and C_2. This method therefore minimizes the 3-D distance between the CS and the reconstructed CS catheter.

Reconstruction of a 3-D volume from bi-plane fluoroscopy is typically a non-trivial problem. In our application, however, the 2-D CS catheter has a very simple and smooth line structure, and hence can be reconstructed straightforwardly using epipolar line constraints, and possibly local line tracing when more than one catheter point intersect with a given epipolar line. Iterative closet point (ICP) based algorithm [18, 19] is used for 3-D/3-D registration between two point sets. Since 3-D/3-D transformation has a close-form solution given the point-to-point correspondence between two point sets, this method typically converges much faster than those iterative optimization methods like Best Neighbor.

2.2. Lasso-Based Motion Compensation

After 2-D/3-D registration between the 3-D volume and the 2-D fluoroscopy using the CS location constraint, as elaborated in the previous section, static overlay can be obtained by overlaying the fluoroscopy with the projected 3-D volume and/or a surface mesh model derived from the 3-D volume using any standard volume/mesh rendering techniques. From this point on, dynamic motion is estimated by tracking the lasso catheter in a mono-plane fluoroscopy to generate a dynamic overlay. For the first frame, semi-automatic 2-D segmentation of the lasso catheter is achieved similarly as the segmentation of the CS catheter, using the method elaborated in Section 2.1. The only difference is that a close-end, instead of an open-end, B-Spline curve is fitted to the 2-D path obtained by Fast Marching, because the lasso-catheter is a circumferential object. The number of control points for the fitted B-spline curve is determined as the ratio of the total length of the original centerline and the pre-defined length for one segment between two neighboring control points.

In the subsequent frames the lasso catheter is tracked automatically by moving the positions of the control points so that the fitted B-Spline curve, denoted by *B*, maximizes the energy *E(B)*:

$$E(B) = \sum_{p=1}^{n} \left(v(p) + \alpha \cdot mc(p) + \beta \cdot \kappa(p) \right) + \sum_{l=1}^{d} r(d) + s(B) \tag{5}$$

here *n* is the number of pixels of the fitted B-Spline curve. For a given pixel *p, v(p)* is the vesselness and hence is maximized for dark tubular structures, and in our case the lasso catheter. *K(p)* is the curvature at pixel *p* and is used to regularize the shape of the tracked lasso catheter. A smoothly-curved shape is preferred over a sharply-curved shape, which confirms to the typical shape of a lasso catheter. The term *mc(p)* is defined as the motion coefficient that represents the appearance change of the current frame from the previous frame at pixel *p*. This term is introduced in order to incorporate the prior knowledge that due to cardiac and respiratory motion the lasso catheter typically moves throughout the fluoroscopic sequence. The relatively static background, such as the spine and/or devices laid on the surface of the body, therefore will be suppressed by this term during the tracking. This makes the tracking algorithm much more robust in the presence of peripheral static dark structures. In addition, this term will not negatively affect the tracking performance even if the motion caused by cardiac and/or respiration is not apparent in certain frames. Wronskian change detector [20] is used to calculate the motion coefficient:

$$\mathrm{mc}(p) - \frac{1}{w} \sum_{j=1}^{w} \left(\frac{I'(p_j)}{I(p_j)} \right)^2 - \frac{1}{w} \sum_{j=1}^{w} \frac{I'(p_j)}{I(p_j)} \tag{6}$$

where *w* is the number of pixels in the neighborhood window of pixel *p* (e.g. *w*=9 for a 3x3 window), p_j is the *j-th* pixel in the neighborhood window of pixel *p*, and I(.) and I'(.) represent the image intensity at the current frame and the previous frame respectively. Wronskian change detector has shown in [20] to be superior to several state-of-the-art motion detectors such as shading model, derivative model, statistical change detection, and linear dependence change detector.

Considering the typical amplitude and the pseudo-cyclic nature of cardiac and respiratory motion, the tracking is further constrained by the term *r(d)* in Equation 5, where *d* is the number of control points of the fitted B-Spline curve. In particular, for a given control point, the changes in its position from both the previous frame and the first frame should be smaller than the corresponding pre-defined thresholds. No penalty is given (i.e. *r(d)* = *0)* if the changes are smaller than their pre-defined thresholds, and a large negative number is assigned (i.e. *r(d)* = *-Inf)* if otherwise. The last term *s(B)* in Equation 5 is to constrain the change in the area of the tracked lasso catheter to be smaller than some threshold, when compared with the lasso catheter segmented from the first frame. Based on Green's Theorem, the area of the tracked lasso catheter is approximated by:

$$S = \frac{1}{2}\sum_{p=1}^{n} X(p)Y(p+1) - X(p+1)Y(p) \tag{7}$$

where $X(p)$ *and* $Y(p)$ are the x and y coordinates of pixel p on the fitted curve B.

During EP fluoroscopic imaging, in order to save X-ray dose it is possible to adopt collimation so that the X-ray exposure is constrained to a small rectangle area instead of the whole image detector. The borders of the collimation area may degrade the tracking performance due to its relatively high image intensity gradient. The borders therefore need to be detected automatically and the searching area for tracking is further constrained to be within the borders. The calculation of the borders is based the one dimensional accumulative intensity profile. For example, to detect the borders in the image width direction (similar calculation applies to the border detection in the image height direction), the intensity profile is calculated as:

$$I_j = \sum_{i=1}^{height} I(p_{ij}) \quad (j = 1\ldots\text{width}) \tag{8}$$

The border in the image width direction is then detected by first finding the position q with the steepest slope (i.e. the largest gradient) in the accumulative intensity profile. The position after q when the intensity increase starts to drop is regarded as the border. In addition, those large intensity gradients in the profile not on the border but caused by image content variation (e.g. the presence of devices) can be excluded by the following ratio, which is much smaller for image content variation than at the true border of the collimation window:

$$I_q \Big/ \frac{1}{q-1}\sum\nolimits_{i=1\ldots q-1} I_i \tag{9}$$

3. EXPERIMENTS

3.1. CS-Based 2-D/3-D Registration

To quantitatively evaluate the performance of our proposed 2-D/3-D registration method using the CS, two experiments were done on simulated data with known ground truth. In the first experiment, the centerline of the CS segmented from a real CT volume was smoothed and elongated to simulate the CS catheter. The simulated CS catheter was then posed with a ground truth transformation and projected onto the two imaging planes to generate the simulated 2-D CS catheters. In the second experiment, some location variations simulating the possible movement of the CS catheter inside the CS was introduced, to investigate its influence on the registration performance of the proposed method. It is assumed that the offset of the catheter from the centerline of the CS due to movement is typically not uniform along the whole catheter. The perturbation therefore was generated by randomly moving the control points of the Cubic B-Spline that fits the simulated catheter. The magnitude of the perturbation was within the range of the half width of a normal CS, i.e. less than 5mm [21]. Two hundred initial starting poses were generated by randomly generating a deviation from the ground truth transformation within the range of -8 to 8 degrees of rotation and -20 to 20 mm of translation in three directions. Several salient points within the distance of 15cm from the CS were chosen to evaluate the registration accuracy.

Table 1 summarizes the registration results for the proposed method on simulated data in both perfect condition and with perturbation. It can be seen that the proposed method was very efficient, accurate, and robust (Figure 1). In addition, random perturbation on the location of the simulated CS catheter did not noticeably affect the registration accuracy for the proposed method, demonstrating the robustness of the proposed method with regard to realistic catheter movement inside the CS.

Table 1. Quantitative evaluation of the performance of CS-based 2-D/3-D registration method on simulated data

	computation time(s)	mean 2D error (mm)	standard deviation 2D error (mm)	Mean 3D error (mm)	standard deviation 3D error (mm)
Experiment I / perfect condition	0.56	1.55	0.08	2.34	0.53
Experiment II / with perturbation	0.62	2.30	0.63	3.19	0.78

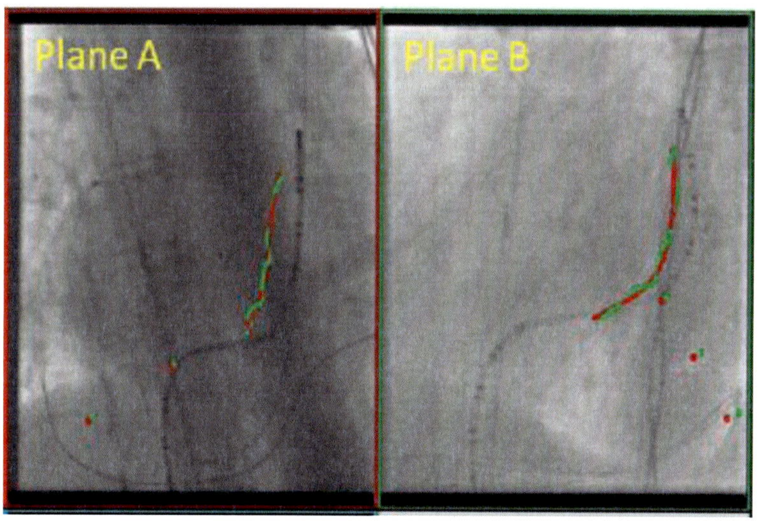

Figure 1. Overlapping of the projected CS (green) and the simulated CS catheter (red) after registration. The three dots represent the salient points used to evaluate the registration accuracy. The results for both plane A (left) and plane B (right) are shown.

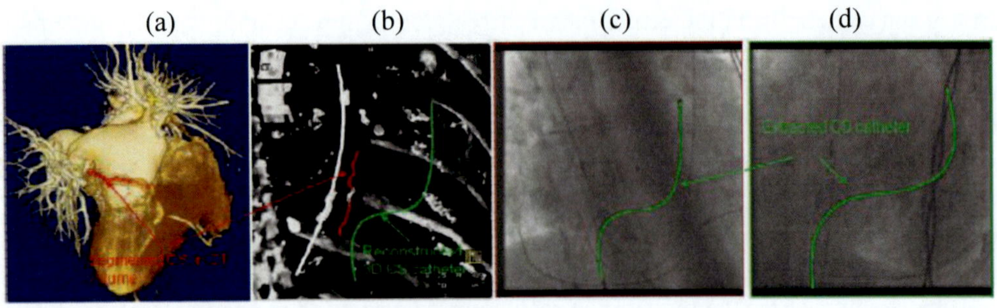

Figure 2. Demonstration of the segmented CS and the reconstructed CS catheter in the CT volume. (a) A CT volume with the CS segmented and highlighted in red. (b) A CT volume showing the segmented CS (red) and the reconstructed CS catheter (green) before registration. (c-d) A segmented CS catheter in the bi-plane fluoroscopic images and highlighted in green.

We further applied our proposed method to *in vivo* clinical data acquired during an EP procedure by a Siemens Axiom Artis dBC biplane system. The CT volume was of size 512 X 512 X 284 and resolution 0.43 X 0.43 X 0.50 mm. The CS in the CT volume and the CS catheter in the bi-plane fluoroscopic images were segmented using the method described in Section 2.1, and the result is shown in Figure 2. The reconstructed 3-D CS catheter is shown in the coordinate of the CT volume to demonstrate its relative position with respect to the CS before registration.

Figure 3 demonstrates the position of the diaphragm and the spine in the 3-D CT volume before and after registration using the proposed method. The contours of the spine and the diaphragm were first outlined from the fluoroscopic image of plane A and then overlaid with the CT volume, in order to demonstrate the registration accuracy of the proposed method.

It is clear that after registration using bi-plane fluoroscopy, the diaphragm and the spine in the CT volume was aligned accurately to those shown in the fluoroscopy. In addition, the trajectory of the 3-D tip of the ablation catheter reconstructed from the biplane fluoroscopy sequences was accurately mapped within the right atrium of the 3-D CT volume after registration, further confirming the registration accuracy.

3.2. Lasso-Based Motion Compensation

We quantitatively evaluated the performance of our proposed lasso catheter tracking algorithm on 13 monoplane fluoroscopic sequences (466 frames) that were acquired during EP procedures on an AXIOM Artis C-arm system (Siemens AG, Healthcare Sector, Forchheim, Germany). To calculate the tracking error, we calculated the average distance of the tracked B-Spline curve to the manual lasso catheter segmentation which was performed under the supervision of a cardiologist. This distance was averaged over all the frames of a particular sequence to arrive at an overall 2-D tracking error for each sequence. The mean average over all the 466 frames was 0.66 ± 0.37 mm. The tracking results on each sequence are summarized in Table 2. An example of image processing steps for tracking the lasso catheter is shown in Figure 4, and several examples of the tracked lasso catheter and the detected border of the collimation window are shown in Figure 5.

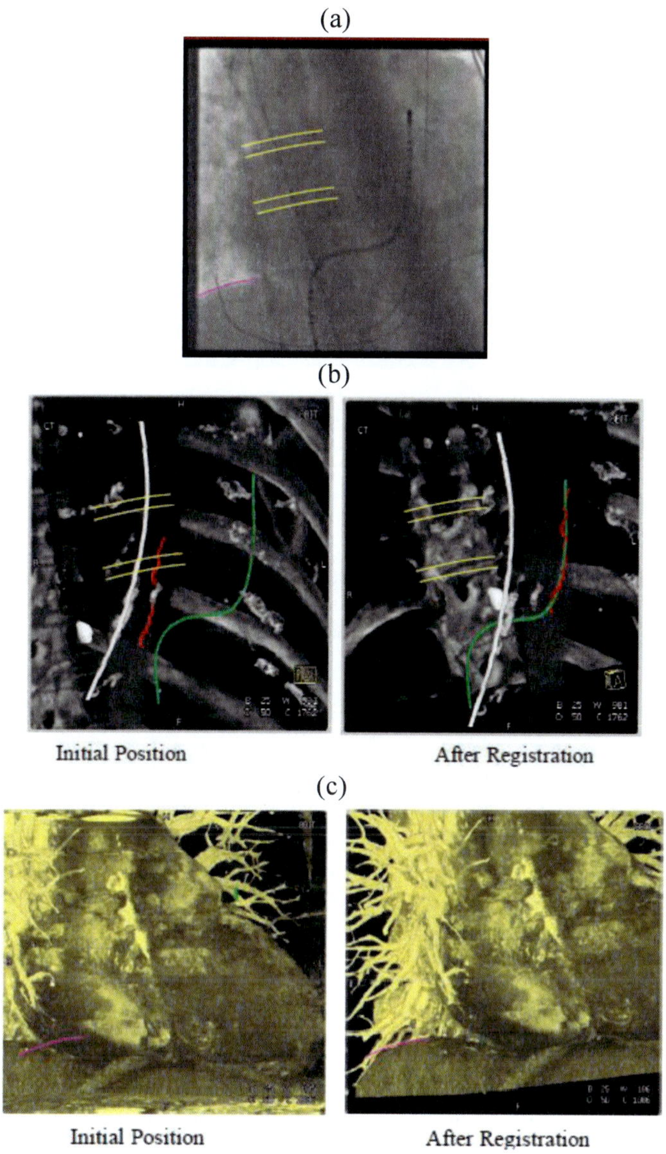

[a] Fluoroscopic image of plane A with the outline of the spine and the diaphragm highlighted.
[b] Overlay of the outline of the spine with the CT volume before (left) and after (right) registration.
[c] Overlay of the outline of the diaphragm with the CT volume before (left) and after (right) registration.

Figure 3. Registration results obtained by the proposed CS-based 2-D/3-D registration method on *in vivo* clinical data.

Table 2. Quantitative evaluation of lasso catheter tracking algorithm on EP fluoroscopic sequences

Sequence	1	2	3	4	5	6	7	8	9	10	11	12	13	Total
# of Frames	23	116	9	10	30	19	18	34	43	38	54	40	32	466
Error (mm)	0.8	0.9	0.7	0.7	0.7	0.6	0.5	0.6	0.4	0.5	0.7	0.4	0.8	0.66
STD (mm)	0.5	0.4	0.5	0.5	0.4	0.4	0.2	0.4	0.2	0.3	0.4	0.3	0.5	0.37

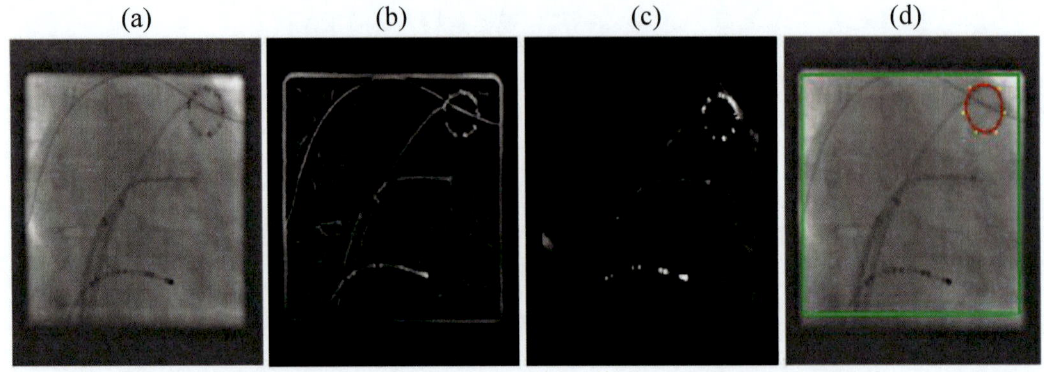

Figure 4. Model-based lasso catheter tracking. a) Original fluoroscopic image b) Vesselness. c) Motion coefficient. It is clear that the spine and the device outside the body have a low motion coefficient, in contrast to the moving lasso and ablation catheters. d) The red curve is the tracked lasso catheter with the control points shown in yellow. The detected borders for X-Ray collimation window are plotted in green.

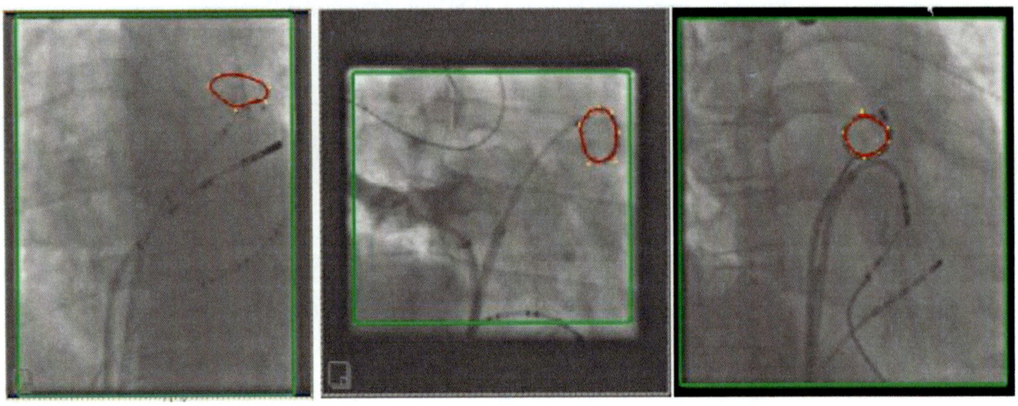

Figure 5. Examples of the tracked lasso catheter and the detected borders of the collimation area.

The tracked lasso catheter can be used for 2-D or 3-D breathing motion compensation on a monoplane setup. For 2-D motion compensation, the 2-D translation and scaling parameters can be approximated directly from the position of the center and the area of the tracked lasso catheter. The estimated translation and scaling parameters then can be used to translate and scale the projection image of the 3-D volume for a dynamic overlay.

Note that 2-D translation only cannot generate very accurate motion compensation due to the fact that breathing motion happens in 3-D, rather than in the imaging plane, and X-ray projection geometry is perspective instead of orthographic.

An illustration is shown in Figure 6, where an ellipse (red) is fitted to the lasso catheter on one fluoroscopic frame (right), and then overlaid onto another frame (left) in the same fluoroscopic sequence after optimal 2-D translation. There is apparent mis-match in scaling due to breathing motion, which can be elegantly corrected by a 3-D rigid-body transformation of the volume (green). 2-D scaling compensation can also remedy the effect of out-of-plane motion and perspective projection on the imaging plane to a certain degree, while real 3-D motion compensation is supposed to be even more accurate (details are given next).

For 3-D motion compensation, a 3-D breathing motion model needs to be built in a training phase. In particular, two fluoroscopic sequences at least 40 degrees apart should be acquired sequentially using a monoplane system, and a 2-D breathing motion trajectory can be generated for each plane by fitting a polynomial to the centers of the tracked lasso catheter for all the ECG-gated frames (Figure 7.a). The 3-D breathing motion trajectory is then reconstructed using the two 2-D breathing motion trajectories from two views by epipolar geometry constraint [22]. During the training phase, deep inhalation and exhalation is recommended in order to cover the largest possible range of patient breathing. In addition, the fluoroscopic sequences should contain a sufficient number of different breathing states during the breathing cycle for a given cardiac phase (say 10 ~ 15 seconds acquisition for each sequence to cover 2 ~ 3 breathing cycles and 10 ~ 15 cardiac cycles).

The reconstructed 3-D motion trajectory represents the 3-D translational motion model of the left atrium (LA) due to respiration at the cardiac phase matching to the 3-D volume (Figure 7.b). In can be seen from Figure 7.b that the displacement of the lasso catheter (and implicitly the displacement of LA) caused by respiratory motion is dominant in cranial-caudal direction, but is also significant in anterior-posterior direction. Motion compensation in the imaging plane only (typically from AP view) as suggested in [11] therefore is not sufficient, especially if the position of the inserting device needs to be localized in the 3-D context of the motion-compensated volumetric data.

After building of the 3-D breathing motion model, the 3-D translational motion of LA due to breathing during EP procedures can be approximated using a monoplane fluoroscopy acquired from any angulations by the following procedures: 1) track the lasso catheter on the monoplane fluoroscopy and calculate the center of the lasso; 2) back-project the center of the tracked lasso catheter according to the imaging geometry; 3) locate the closest intersection of the back-projection ray to the constructed 3-D motion trajectory to get the motion estimate; 4) the 3-D motion estimate is then applied to the static fluoroscopic overlay by moving the 3-D volume correspondingly. This way, we can obtain an animated version of our initial static overlay that moves in sync with the real anatomy (Figure 8).

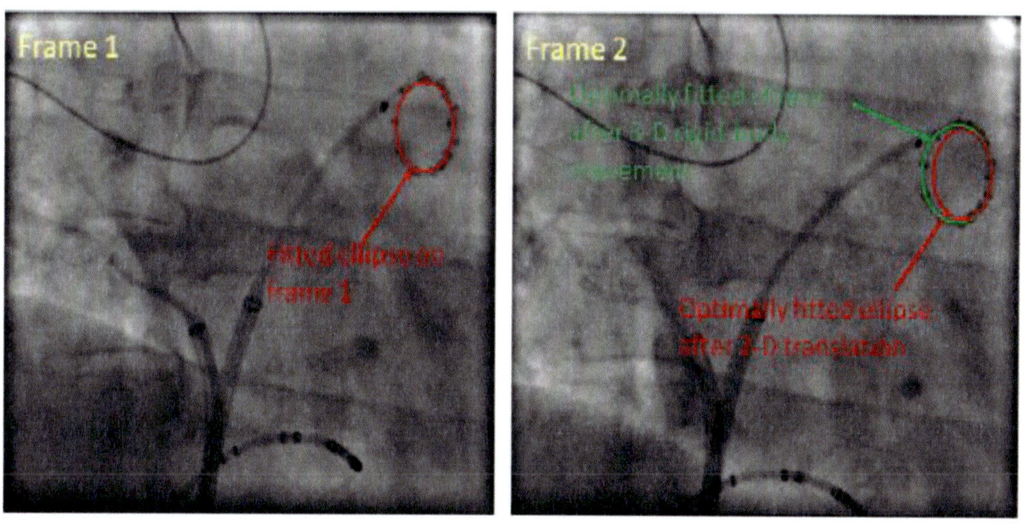

Figure 6. An example of scaling effect on 2-D fluoroscopic images due to breathing.

(a) (b)

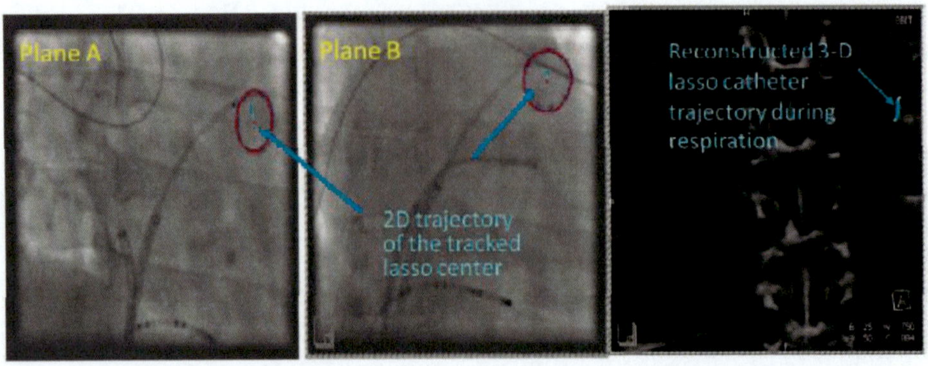

Figure 7. Illustration of motion compensation using the tracked lasso catheter. (a) Lasso catheter tracking on ECG-gated frames from two monoplane views. The red dot is the center of the tracked lasso catheter for the current frame. The 2-D motion trajectory of the centers of the tracked lasso catheter throughout the sequence is plotted in cyan. (b) The reconstructed 3-D respiratory motion trajectory of the center of the tracked lasso catheter during the breathing cycle is shown in the relative position to the 3-D volumetric spine from the AP view.

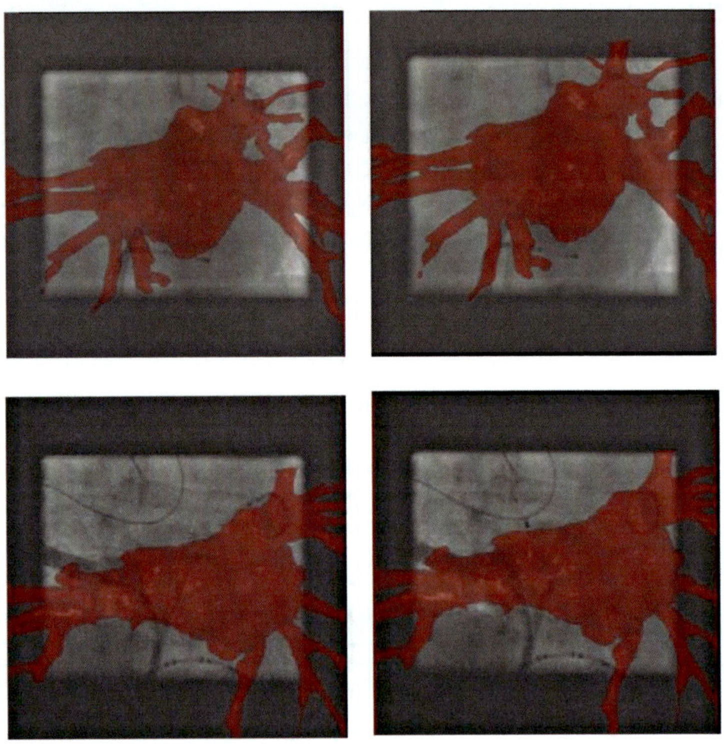

Figure 8. Two examples (one example in each row) of motion compensation for the overlay of fluoroscopic sequence with a surface model of left atrium and pulmonary veins. One frame of a non-motion compensated sequence with fluoroscopic overlay is shown in the left image, where the lasso catheter is outside the left atrium in the static overlay due to respiratory motion. The same frame with motion compensation is shown in the right image. Note that the lasso catheter and the contrast agent are now matched to the morphology of the LA and PVs after motion compensation.

CONCLUSION

Existing 2-D/3-D registration techniques typically require that the vessels of interest in fluoroscopy be opacified by injecting contrast agent into the patient [23]. Without the contrast agent to highlight the vessels, intensity and feature-based 2-D/3-D registration in a robust manner is extremely difficult with the existing approaches. For landmark-based registration, accurate manual picking of 3-D points on the volumetric CT data could be laborious and prone to errors, and it is not always possible to identify the corresponding landmarks in the 2-D fluoroscopy without highlighting the region of interest via contrast agent, because those clearly visible structures in the fluoroscopy, such as catheters and other devices, are usually not present in the pre-operative 3-D volumes.

This chapter describes a 2-D/3-D registration technique for EP procedures that does not need additional contrast agent administration. Registration was done by optimizing the location constraint between the anatomical pathways (vessels) that catheter goes through or is placed. Since CS is relatively narrow and has clear bending (not a straight line), the registration can be highly accurate, and the capture range of the proposed method is much larger than that of the conventional intensity-based 2-D/3-D registration. Similar work has been presented in [24], where the CT volume was registered to mono-plane fluoroscopic images by aligning the superior vena cava (SVC) and the CS with a catheter placed inside the CS via SVC. However, registration using mono-plane fluoroscopic image can produce significant errors in the depth direction, meaning that although the projected 2-D displacement is small, registration error in 3-D can be indeed substantially larger. Utilization of bi-plane fluoroscopy dramatically increases the registration accuracy in 3-D, especially when there are rotation errors. In addition, SVC is typically wider than CS, providing a less accurate location constraint than CS, and potentially more difficult to segment. Another limitation of the method proposed in [24] is that registration is accomplished mainly through manual adjustment, especially for correction of rotation errors, which is laborious, error-prone, and the performance varies among users.

We further developed a novel method for 3-D breathing motion compensation for EP procedures using a monoplane system. The proposed method for lasso catheter tracking is based on a close-end B-spline model constructed from the first frame. Compared to template-based method, model-based method is more robust to possible appearance changes, e.g. caused by injection of contrast agent and presence of other moving device. In addition, template-based method typically suffers from drifting issue due to the need to update the template from previous tracking results with accumulative tracking errors. The proposed algorithm is specifically designed for tracking the lasso catheter in EP fluoroscopic images by utilizing motion coefficients and automatic detection of the X-ray collimation window. Our experiments on clinical EP fluoro sequences show that the tracking error averages at 0.66 ± 0.37 mms, and no apparent drifting is observed. Considering that breathing motion shown in typical EP fluoroscopic images is in the range of 15mm and for some patients can be up to 40mm for deep breathing, our method has the potential to significantly improve the accuracy of 3-D overlay for EP navigation.

The proposed method offers several advantages. First, bi-plane fluoroscopy is needed only at the beginning of the procedure, for the purpose of 2-D/3-D registration and optionally construction of the patient-specific 3-D breathing motion model. Dynamic motion compensation is then performed in 2-D or 3-D on a monoplane system, which is both accurate and cost effective with the minimized radiation, compared to a biplane system. Second, to perform registration and motion estimation, we utilize commonly available EP catheters, i.e. the CS catheter and the ring-shaped lasso catheter. Since these devices are often used for PV ablations, it is workflow-friendly and does not require fiducial markers or additional contrast agent to be administered. Third, during the isolation of the four pulmonary veins during AF ablation, the lasso catheter is typically fixed at the ostium of the PV that is to be ablated. By tracking the lasso catheter, we can obtain a motion estimate right at the ablation site. Therefore motion estimation and compensation is essentially done in one step. Fourth, there are no restrictions for the 3-D data set that can be used as a fluoroscopic overlay. In other words, the 3-D data set could come from MRI, CT or C-arm CT, e.g., syngo DynaCT Cardiac (Siemens AG, Healthcare Sector, Forchheim, Germany).

Acknowledgments

The author is grateful to all the past and present colleagues for their insightful discussion and indispensable contributions to the work presented here, and thankful to Siemens Corporate Research for providing the platform to perform the interesting research presented in this chapter.

References

[1] B. Gage, A. Waterman, W. Shannon, M. Boechler, M. Rich, and M. Radford, "Validation of Clinical Classification Schemes for Predicting Stroke," *Journal of the American Medical Association*, vol. 285, no. 22, pp. 2864–2870, June 2001.

[2] M. Haissaguerre, L. Gencel, B. Fischer, P. L. Metayer, F. Poquet, F. I. Marcus, and J. Clementy, "Successful catheter ablation of atrial fibrillation," *Journal of Cardiovascular Electrophysiology*, vol. 5, no. 12, pp. 1045–1052, December 1994.

[3] H. Calkins, J. Brugada, D. Packer, R. Cappato, S. Chen, H. Crijns, R. Damiano, D. Davies, D. Haines, M. Haissaguerre, Y. Iesaka, W. Jackman, P. Jais, H. Kottkamp, K. Kuck, B. Lindsay, F. Marchlinski, P. McCarthy, J. Mont, F. Moradi, K. Nademanee, A. Natale, C. Pappone, E. Prystowsky, A. Raviele, J. Ruskin, and R. Shemin, "HRS/EHRA/ECAS Expert Consensus Statement on Catheter and Surgical Ablation of Atrial Fibrillation: Recommendations for Personnel, Policy, Procedures and Follow-Up," *Europace*, vol. 9, no. 6, pp. 335–379, June 2007.

[4] O. Wazni, N. Marrouche, D. Martin, A. Verma, M. Bhargava, W. Saliba, D. Bash, R. Schweikert, J. Brachmann, J. Gunther, K. Gutleben, E. Pisano, D. Potenza, R. Fanelli, A. Raviele, S. Themistoclakis, A. Rossillo, A. Bonso, and A. Natale, "Radiofrequency ablation vs antiarrhythmic drugs as first-line treatment of symptomatic atrial fibrillation: a randomized trial," *Journal of the American Medical Association*, vol. 293, no. 21, pp. 2634–2640, January 2005.

[5] R. Cappato, H. Calkins, S.-A. Chen, W. Davies, Y. Iesaka, J. Kalman, Y.-H. Kim, G. Klein, D. Packer, and A. Skanes, "Worldwide Survey on the Methods, Efficacy, and

Safety of Catheter Ablation for Human Atrial Fibrillation," *Circulation*, vol. 111, pp. 1100–1105, February 2005.

[6] R. Liao, "2-D/3-D Registration Of Computed Tomographic Volumes with Fluoroscopic Images By Spines For EP Applications", IEEE *International Symposium on Biomedical Imaging: From Nano to Macro* 2010; 1213-1216.

[7] A. Brost, R. Liao, J. Hornegger, N. Strobel, "3-D Respiratory Motion Compensation during EP Procedures by Image-based 3-D Lasso Catheter Model Generation and Tracking", *Med. Image Comput. Comput. Assist. Interv.* 2009, vol.12, pp. 394-401.

[8] A. Brost, R. Liao, J. Hornegger, N. Strobel, "Respiratory Motion Compensation by Model-Based Catheter Tracking during EP Procedures", *Medical Image Analysis* 2010; 14(5):695-706.

[9] K. Rhode, et al., "Evaluation of the use of multimodality skin markers for the registration of pre-procedure cardiac MR images and intra-procedure x-ray fluoroscopy images for image guided cardiac electrophysiology procedures", *SPIE* 2008.

[10] H. Timinger, S. Krueger, K. Dietmayer, J. Borgert, "Motion Compensated Coronary Interventional Navigation by Means of Diaphram Tracking and Elastic Motion Models", *Physics in Medicine and Biology* 2005; 50(3):491–503.

[11] S. Atasoy, et. al., "Real-time Respiratory Motion Tracking: Roadmap Correction for Hepatic Artery Catheterizations", *Proc. SPIE* 6918, 1-9(2008).

[12] Ross, et al., "Motion Correction for Augmented Fluoroscopy - Application to Liver Embolization ", *Proc. ISBI*, 1553-1556(2008).

[13] J. Ector, etc., "Changes in Left Atrial Anatomy Due to Respiration: Impact on Three-Dimensional Image Integration during Atrial Fibrillation Ablation", *Journal of Cardiovascular Electrophysiology* 19(8), 828-834(2008).

[14] A. Frangi, W. Niessen, K. Vincken, and M. Viergever, "Multiscale Vessel Enhancement Filtering", *Lecture Notes in Computer Science*, vol. 1496, pp.130-137, 1998.

[15] E. N. Mortensen. W. A. Barrett, "Intelligent Scissors for Image Composition", ACM, 1995.

[16] J. A. Sethian, "Level Set Methods and Fast Marching Methods: Evolving Interfaces in Computational Geometry, Fluid Mechanics", *Computer Vision and Material Sciences*, Cambridge University Press, second edition, 1998.

[17] S. Sauer. "An Optimized Algorithm for Coronary Sinus Segmentation in MSCT Datasets", Diploma Thesis, University of Karlsruhe, Germany. 2005.

[18] J. Feldmar, N. Ayache, F. Betting, "3D-2D projective registration of free-form curves and surfaces", *Computer Vision and Image Understanding*. 65(3): 403-424, 1997.

[19] P. Besl, N. Mckay, "A method for Registration of 3-D Shapes", *IEEE Transaction on Pattern Analysis and Machine Intelligence*, 14(2): 239-256, 1992.

[20] E. Durucan, T. Ebrahimi, "Change Detection and Background Extraction by Linear Algebra", *IEEE Proc.* 89, 1368-1381(2001).

[21] J. Doig, J. Saito, L. Harris, E. Downar. "Coronary Sinus Morphology in Patients with Atrioventricular Junctional Reentry Tachycardia and Other Supraventricular Tachyarrhythmias", *Circulation*. 92:436-441, 1995.

[22] R. Hartley and A. Zisserman, "Multiple View Geometry", Cambridge University Press, 2003.

[23] R. Liao, C. Guetter, C. Xu, Y. Sun, A. Khamene, F. Sauer, "Learning-Based 2D/3D Rigid Registration Using Jensen-Shannon Divergence for Image-Guided Surgery", 228-235, MIAR 2006.

[24] J. Sra, D. Krum, A. Malloy, M. Vass, B. Belanger, E. Soubelet, R. Vaillant, M. Akhtar, "Registration of Three-dimensional Left Atrial Computed Tomographic images with Projection Images Obtained Using Fluoroscopy", *Circulation.* 112(24):3677-9, 2005.

In: New Developments in Angiography Research
Editors: K. I. Sanders and A. M. Jackson
ISBN: 978-1-62081-492-5

Chapter IV

ADVANCES IN NEURO-ANGIOGRAPHY

Nader Sawiris and Shyam Prabhakaran
Department of Neurological Sciences, Rush University Medical Center
Chicago, IL, US

ABSTRACT

Angiography is a term which describes different techniques used to visualize the blood vessels. Computed tomography angiography, magnetic resonant angiography, and digital subtraction angiography are the vascular techniques commonly used for this purpose. These procedures are typically used to diagnose vascular abnormalities such as cerebral aneurysms, arteriovenous malformations and fistulas, cerebral vasospasm, intracranial stenosis, and vasculitis. Catheter angiography and computed tomography angiography (CTA) as well as magnetic resonance angiography (MRA) have progressively improved in the past several decades. In many situations, the noninvasive angiographic methods may be equal to catheter angiography for diagnostic accuracy. In other circumstances, conventional angiogram remains the gold standard for diagnosis of many vessel abnormalities and pathology. However, in many conditions a combination of more than one technique is reasonable and warranted for better evaluation of the vascular abnormalities. In this review, we will discuss some of the recent developments in angiography research and will provide updates on the new techniques in CTA, MRA, and DSA in diagnosis cerebrovascular abnormalities.

INTRODUCTION

Angiography is a term, which describes various imaging modalities used to visualize the blood vessels. Computed tomography angiography (CTA), magnetic resonance angiography (MRA) and digital subtraction angiography (DSA) are several vascular imaging techniques used for this purpose. In the field of stroke, these procedures are typically used to diagnose vascular abnormalities and diseases such as cerebral aneurysms, arteriovenous malformations, cerebral vasospasm, intracranial stenosis, and vasculitis. Each technique has progressively improved in the past several decades.

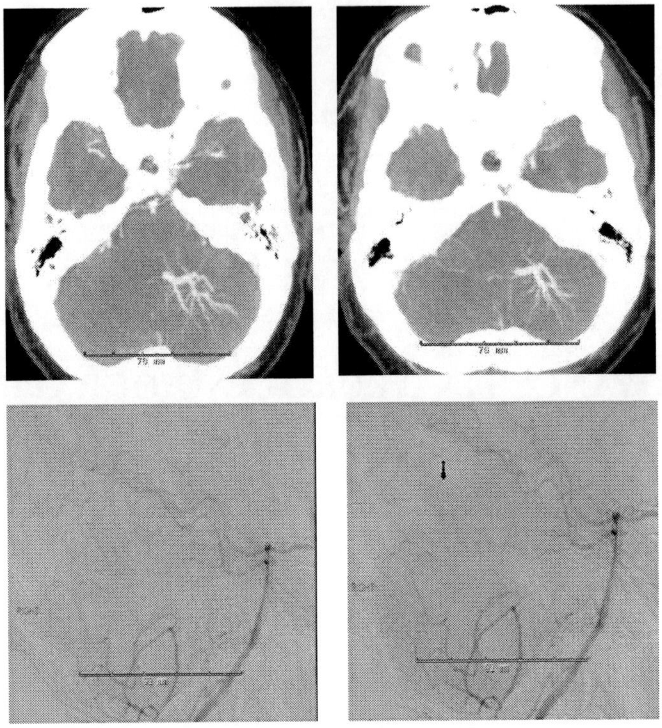

Figure 1. 54 year old woman with past medical history of depression and hypertension presented with sudden onset of vertigo with nausea and vomiting. Symptoms were positional vertigo but further imaging (CTA-top) revealed abnormal finding that was concerning for arteriovenous malformation. Cerebral angiogram (bottom) for further evaluation revealed large cerebellar venous angioma with drainage into the deep venous system. The patient symptomatically improved with meclizine and anti-emetics and was discharged home after reassurance.

In many situations, the noninvasive angiographic methods may equal catheter angiography for diagnostic accuracy. [1] Furthermore, these noninvasive imaging tools have the advantage of avoiding patient exposure to the potential neurologic complications associated with the catheter angiography.

Non-invasive modalities have recently demonstrated satisfactory spatial resolution within 2 to 3 mm, a level adequate to diagnose various clinical neurovascular conditions [2,3,4,5]

On the other hand, in many circumstances conventional angiogram remains the gold standard. This is partly because the aforementioned non-invasive techniques do not offer the temporal resolution advantage, which makes them inefficient in showing early venous filling in arteriovenous shunt or visualizing feeding and draining vascular patterns [6]. In some cases, DSA is necessary to exclude anomalies like AVMs that were suggested on CTA (Figure 1). In many situations, however, a combination of more than one technique is reasonable and warranted for better evaluation of vascular abnormalities. Satoh et al. [7] reported that integration of data obtained by different diagnostic tools including 3D-MR and CT angiography may improve peri-operative assessment of the vascular cerebral aneurysms. *Inoue et al.* [8] reported that, for diagnostic purposes and for planning for treatment, using other imaging technique like 3D-CTA preceding DSA is beneficial in selective catheterization of arteries at some spinal levels. In this chapter, we will discuss some of the recent developments in angiography research and will provide new updates on the new techniques in DSA, CTA, and MRA in the diagnosis of cerebrovascular disease.

DIGITAL SUBTRACTION ANGIOGRAPHY (DSA)

Digital subtraction angiography (DSA) is an interventional technique used to interrogate the cerebral vasculature and allows endovascular treatment of some conditions. It uses fluoroscopy to visualize injected contrasts as they opacify target blood vessels. [9] Images are then digitized by means of software to remove the pre-contrast background image in order to generate images of contrast-filled vessels. Catheter cerebral angiography has advanced considerably since its first use in humans in 1927. [10,11] Since the 1990s, there has been a great evolution of DSA due to the introduction of 3D rotational angiography, which can be used to produce a 3D replica of the images. [9] Angiography, which was first introduced by neurologists [12], is now done by radiologists and neurosurgeons, as well as interventional neurologists.

The most common indications for DSA are the diagnosis of aneurysms and arteriovenous malformations, venous diseases, pre-operative management of meningiomas, diagnosis and treatment of arterial stroke including acute ischemic stroke, cerebral vasospasm, intracranial stenosis, and vasculitis. [1] Furthermore, intra-operative angiography has been progressively applied in the surgical management of cerebral aneurysms and arteriovenous malformations. This is done with few complications [13,14] and can assist in providing definitive combination therapies for complex neurovascular conditions.

Catheter cerebral angiogram, which was considered a very risky procedure in its infancy, now is considered relatively safe if done by experienced operators. The first few patients who underwent this procedure developed different complications ranging from transient events like aphasia to more severe ones like Horner syndrome related to contrast material to the most dreadful complication, death from thromboembolism or vessel perforation.[15] Moreover, the Thorotrast, which was introduced in 1931 as a contrast material, was found to induce malignancies.[16] Now, with safer techniques and agents, studies have shown complication rates are as low as 0.3%. These complications are mostly related to the utilization of arterial closure devices and more common in those over 65 years of age. [1,17] Commons complications include puncture site hematomas, contrast-related nephropathy, ischemic stroke, and the risk of vessel perforation during interventions. However, all risks should be carefully considered in each patient with the goal of appropriate patient selection and adverse event prevention.

In light of this, some authors believe that the use of DSA for diagnostic purposes will possibly diminish especially with the increasing accuracy of other non-invasive methods. [18] The need for catheter angiography will always exist because of its unique role in determining the nature of dynamic lesions such as AVMs and the increasing use of endovascular therapies for cerebrovascular disease. [9] Despite the debate in literature on the best methods for vascular imaging, there is consensus that DSA remains the diagnostic gold standard. [19,20,21,22,23] In a study to support this, *Nishimura et al.* [24]reported that the usefulness of conventional MRI, time-of-flight MRA, and contrast-enhanced MRA in evaluating feeding arteries and tumor stain in head and neck is limited. DSA offers incomparable spatial and temporal resolution that helps to identify the feeding arteries and gives accurate data regarding the tumor vascularity. Vessel selectivity is another advantage that makes cerebral angiography unmatched with regard to accuracy and extent of diagnostic information offered [15] Finally, with the addition of 3D rendering, DSA combines both the advantages of fine anatomic and temporal imaging with the 3D imaging capabilities available with CTA or MRA [25,26,27,28] With this achievement, 3D-DSA has acquired a major role in decision making and treatment planning by providing a very thorough detailed anatomical information with very high resolution prior to intervention. [29]

One of the weaknesses of cerebral angiography is the inability of 3D-DSA to concurrently picture bony and vascular anatomy, an notable advantage of CT angiography [30,31,32] However, *Gailloud et al.* [25] describe a new 3D digital angiography (DA) reconstruction algorithm that permits simultaneous imaging of the osseous and vascular structures obtained through a rotational cerebral angiogram. Both modalities of reconstruction, 3D-DSA and 3D-DA, can be achieved with a single injection of contrast material. This new algorithm combines the advantages of DSA and some of that of CTA. It permits 3D-DA to integrate the spatial resolution of 3D-DSA with the topographic bony findings readily available by CT angiography. However, some limitations remain: the inability to obtain good images and fine anatomical details of aneurysms and small perforator vessels which neighbor bony structures [31,32] *Gailloud et al.* [33] further defined another algorithm for rotational angiography that incorporates reconstructions of the blood vessels and the bony structures in a 3D image. This new algorithm, called three-dimensional fusion digital subtraction angiography (FDSA), is based on split renderings of the mask and contrast sequences. The two 3D image sets, 3D-bone and 3D-digital subtraction angiography, are merged into one 3-dimensional image. It offers high-resolution images of vascular and body structures, promotes the role of conventional angiography in illustrating the cranial vascular pathology, especially those at the skull base, and helps in surgical planning.

Color-coded DSA is another potential application that is being studied and may be of great use in the future given the useful diagnostic information that it can provide. [34,35]In 1986, *Hunter et al.* [36] introduced a technique to obtain physiologic data by using time-attenuation curves as a means of obtaining reliable measures of organ perfusion. Using parametric color-coding to offer functional information and quantification of perfusion, it can differentiate areas that are over- or under-perfused and assess antegrade and collateral perfusion blood flow and blood volume. This new emerging technique could offer information that can match real-time quantitative perfusion, currently available from CT perfusion imaging. Such data may be useful to detect impairment of blood supply to the brain (e.g. acute ischemic stroke, intracranial stenosis, and Moyamoya syndrome) in real-time and to monitor responses to interventions. This technique may be superior to CT perfusion in that it avoids the risks of additional radiation exposure. [37] *Strother et al.* [38] conducted a study to observe the effects of a color-coding algorithm on the reading of 2D-DSA and showed that the color-coded DSA made findings more obvious, without the need for additional doses of radiation or contrast dye. They also reported that in more than 20% of cases studied, the new findings significantly guided treatment planning. Arteriovenous anomalies are other scenarios which may benefit from parametric color coding through the ability to display arterial feeders and abnormal veins.

Computed Tomography Angiography (CTA)

Computed tomography angiography (CTA) visualizes the lumen of blood vessels using x-ray radiation and injected iodinated contrast. These images can be reconstructed to create a 3-D image. The use of CTA for the diagnosis of intracranial vascular abnormalities has increased in the past decade. It is viewed as a standard technique for the detection of cerebral aneurysms with an improving sensitivity that is at this moment very close to that of DSA. For instance, it has been used as a helpful diagnostic tool, in addition to DSA when diagnostic angiogram is unrevealing. [39] CTA can also be used in the acute setting of aneurysmal subarachnoid hemorrhage for early critical decision-making and obviates the need for DSA in many cases. [40] CTA has also proved to be reliable in offering sufficient data such as in the pre-operative assessment of intracranial aneurysms. [41] A recent study observed that decisions to treat ruptured aneurysms in the anterior circulation may be made based on CTA findings alone. [42] With the improvement of 3D-CTA, it can spare patients the risks of DSA. It allows clear visualization of the lesions and allow for operative planning. For intracranial stenosis, CTA compared favorably with DSA with high sensitivity and specificity. [43]

One of the advantages of CTA is the ability to provide anatomic relationships of structures and tissue surrounding vascular lesions, which is very helpful in making operative decision-making and planning. [8] This is particularly true of vessel-bone interfaces. The sensitivity of CTA for detection of cerebral aneurysms ≤ 5 mm near the skull base is believed to be better that DSA. [44] One of the applications of 3D-CTA is the ability to eliminate bony structures which may obscure vascular lesions at the skull base. [45]In a comparison of 46 patients who underwent CTA and DSA for diagnosis of intracranial aneurysm, CTA performed very similarly to DSA and required lower radiation doses. [46] However, very small aneurysms (< 3mm) may be missed (Figure 2).

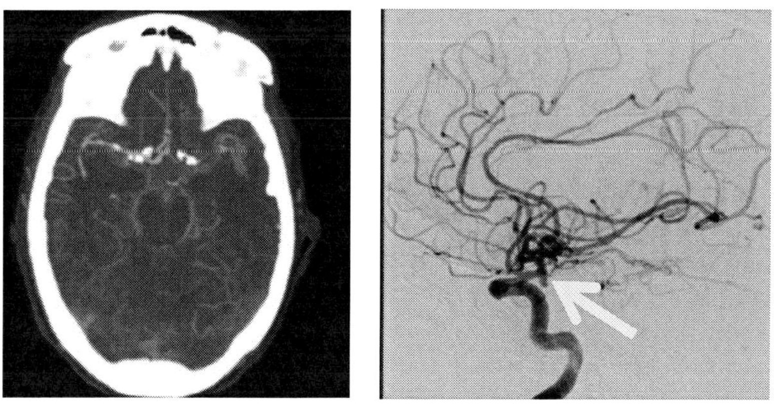

Figure 2. 76-year-old woman with hypertension who presented with headache and dizziness. CTA (top) did not reveal any aneurysm. Cerebral angiogram (bottom) for further evaluation showed right posterior communicating artery aneurysm (3 x 3mm).

CTA technology continues to evolve and improve. Spatial resolution is one major area that has witnessed enhancements. [2,3,4,5] However, lack of temporal resolution remains one of the main limitations of CTA, which is a well-known strength of DSA. This makes it inadequate in the diagnosis of vascular lesions like small AVMs. One of the emerging techniques to overcome this limitation is time-resolved CTA (4D-CTA). [47,48] This technique offers dynamic analysis of blood flow. *Willems et al.* [6] conducted a study on whole head 4D-CTA to evaluate its use for AVM diagnosis and follow-up. In 17 patients with untreated AVMs who underwent DSA imaging as well as 4D-CTA, 4D-CTA was able to spot all AVMs using cross-sectional and perfusion images though the nidus size was underestimated in four cases.

Another addition in the generations of CT scanners is the multi-detector CT. This utilizes the same principle of CT but with multiple rows of detectors, which allows for faster scanning with greater coverage and better spatial and temporal resolution. [49,50] Multi-detector CTA (MD-CTA) is also termed multi-detector array helical CT, multi-channel CT, and multi-slice CT. In a study conducted by *Kato et al.* [51]to evaluate the usefulness of MD-CTA versus standard single slice CTA and DSA in cases with cerebral aneurysm, MD-CTA better appreciated cerebral aneurysms and provided enough detail for surgical planning. One of the advantages of the shorter scanning time is the ability to use less volume of contrast material without compromise in detail. [52,53] In another study using MD-CTA, *Tamaura et al.* [54] demonstrated that with the use of 16-MDCT 3D angiography, contrast material can be reduced from 100 mL to 50 mL. This has many benefits such as cost reductions and decreased risk of contrast nephropathy.

Magnetic Resonance Angiography (MRA)

With the widespread use of magnetic resonance imaging in the past decade, MRA has become a commonly employed non-invasive technique to visualize blood vessels. MRA is done with or without the use of contrast enhanced angiographic techniques. Non-contrast MR angiographic techniques have been used more frequently though contrast-enhanced MRA (CE-MRA) are gaining popularity. Time-of-flight and phase contrast (PC) are the typical methods used of the non-contrast MRA techniques. Time-of-flight (TOF) MRA detects flow in the lumen of blood vessels based on visualizing the magnetic resonance of blood and does not rely on opacification of the lumen of the vessels as in DSA or CTA. As such, it is prone to over-estimating stenosis and poorly distinguishes trickle-flow from complete occlusion. This is overcome with the use of CE-MRA. Although considered safer than iodinated contrast, it should be noted that gadolinium dye has been recently associated with nephrogenic systemic fibrosis. [55,56]

Overall, MRA is considered a safe non-invasive imaging technique. One of its advantages over CTA is that it does not involve any exposure to ionizing radiation. On the other hand, disadvantages of MRA are its higher cost, vulnerability to movement artifact, and lengthy acquisition time making it less attractive in emergency situations. MRI is contraindicated in patients with pacemaker or foreign metallic implants and may be limited in patients who are severely claustrophobic. Finally, gadolinium-enhanced MRA carries risks in patient suffering from kidney disease.

Over the years, MRA has developed considerably. Inadequate sensitivity of MRA improved with the introduction of 3Tesla magnetic field, making it capable of detecting unruptured aneurysms < 3 mm with a sensitivity of about 85–93% and 93–97% in aneurysms

> 3 mm in size. [57] Monitoring of aneurysm recanalization after coiling is one of the new applications of MRA, where using MRA with 3D-TOF or CE-MRA proved to be a great benefit. TOF-MRA may substitute for DSA, [58] avoiding its invasive and procedural risks and is sometimes an alternative to CTA, avoiding the exposure to radiation and the risks associated with iodinated contrast dye. However, it is more challenging to diagnose in-stent stenosis or the completeness of coil embolization on 3D TOF-MRA due to susceptibility artifact produced from the intracranial stent (i.e signal loss at the stented segment of the parent artery). [59,60] In a study aiming at the evaluation of the value of follow up CE-MRA and 3D TOF-MRA in 5 cases where the Enterprise stent was placed for management of intracranial aneurysm, *Takayama et al.* [61] compared the visualization of the parent artery lumen and the aneurysm neck in 3D TOF-MRA and CE-MRA against DSA. In all 5 cases, 3D TOF-MRA failed to clearly visualize the parent artery lumen as well as the aneurysm neck due to stent artifacts. However, CE-MRA was able to adequately confirm parent artery lumen and aneurysm neck with the same accuracy as DSA. However, in another study aimed at comparing the ability of CE-MRA and 3D TOF-MRA to detect residual neck and aneurysm reperfusion after coil embolization for cerebral aneurysms, no significant advantage of CE-MRA over 3D TOF-MRA was observed. [62]

Although CE-MRA could overcome some of the disadvantages faced by TOF-MRA, CE-MRA also has some pitfalls that limit its use in assessing for in-stent stenosis or recanalization of brain aneurysms that was treated with stent-assisted coil embolization. One of those disadvantages is the enhancement of the walls of the aneurysm that can be interpreted falsely as recanalization or stenosis. [63] An application recently used in an attempt to overcome this weakness is time-resolved 3D contrast-enhanced MRA (4D-MRA). This technique appears to be effective for follow-up of aneurysms after stent-assisted coil embolization. In addition, it has been used to diagnose lesions such as AVMs and stenosis. In 4D-MRA, appreciation of the arterial and venous phases is obtained by subtraction of the first image which acts as the mask image [63,64,65] thus competing with DSA for the diagnosis of these lesions.

4D-MRA has been shown to be helpful in pre- and post-operative evaluation of cranial AVMs. *Hadizadeh et al.* compared results of 4D-MRA with that of DSA in 56 patients with AVMs and found that 4D-MRA can provide reliable results that can be used in the post-operative follow-up based on its high spatial and temporal resolution. [66] *Choi et al.* [63] conducted a study to compare the use of the 4D-MRA with that of 3D TOF-MRA and DSA after stent-assisted coil embolization for intracranial aneurysms, observing significantly better quality images obtained by 4D-MRA with all types of stents when compared with that of 3D TOF-MRA. A recent study by Lim et al. [67] concluded that 4D-MRA at 3.0 T is very useful in detecting residual AVMs after gamma-knife radiosurgery with sensitivities of 64-80% and specificities of 91-100%. Given the limited sensitivity, improvement in this technique is warranted before it could replace conventional angiography for residual AVM detection. A major disadvantage of MRA and CTA techniques is the distortion of the images by stent or coil artifact. DSA has been, therefore, the test of choice in these instances. Quantitative magnetic resonance angiography (QMRA) is a promising technique to overcome the limitation of MRA in diagnosing intracranial in-stent stenosis. [68]It involves the combination of TOF-MRA and PC-MRA [69] and allows for quantifying arterial blood flow in addition to showing vascular anatomy. Thus, stenosis detection is based on change in flow rather than relying on the anatomy which is usually distorted by the artifact of the stent.

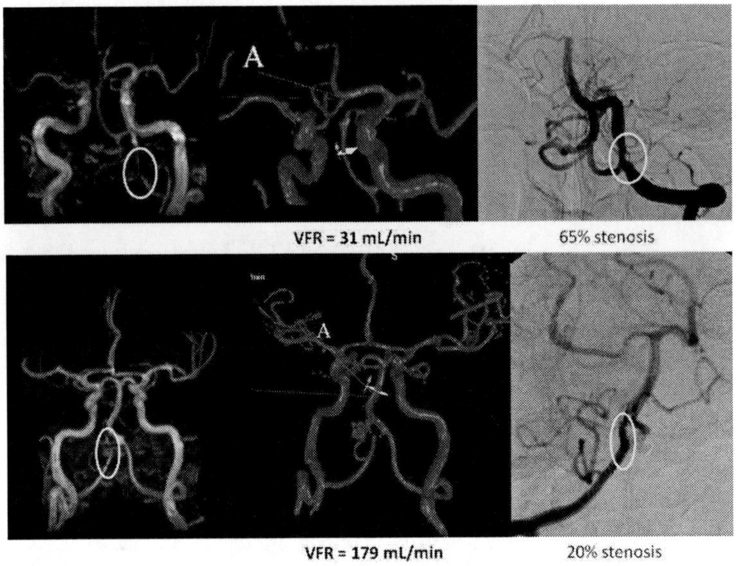

Figure 3. Top-Vertebral artery (VA) stent with flow gap due to artifact on TOF-MRA, QMRA shows normal volumetric flow rate and DSA confirms no in-stent stenosis; Bottom-VA stent with flow gap on TOF-MRA, QMRA shows decreased volumetric flow rate and DSA confirms in-stent-stenosis.

Table. Advantages and disadvantages of DSA, CTA and MRA with examples of new emerging concepts to improve diagnostic capabilities

	Advantages	Disadvantages	New emerging concepts
DSA	- Temporal resolution - Spatial resolution - Vessel selectivity - Intervention	- Invasive procedure with risks - Not always available on emergent basis - Not widely available - Radiation risks - Contrast risks	- 3D digital angiography (DA) reconstruction algorithm - Three-dimensional fusion digital subtraction angiography (FDSA) - Color-coded DSA
CTA	- Non invasive - Available in most emergency rooms - Rapid acquisition	- Lack of temporal resolution - Radiation risks - Contrast risks - Bone and metal artifacts	- 4D-CTA - Multi-detector CT
MRA	- Non invasive - No radiation risks - Vessel wall and soft-tissue imaging	- Higher cost - Longer acquisition time - Prone to movement and metallic artifacts - Contraindicated in cases with pacemakers, foreign metallic bodies and claustrophobia - Gadolinium risks - Lacks temporal resolution	- 3Tesla or higher magnets - 4D-MRA - QMRA

Prabhakaran et al. [68] studied 14 patients and found that all cases that had decreased blood flow in the intracranial stent on QMRA scan also had in-stent stenosis confirmed by the DSA and all patients with normal QMRA did not have significant in-stent stenosis on DSA (Figure 3). Another study using QMRA confirmed that it may be a reliable non-invasive method to identify restenosis in patients who underwent stenting for intracranial stenosis. [70] A > 25% reduction in flow on QMRA may indicate restenosis of an intracranial stent. Lastly, a study in patients with intracranial (Wingspan) stents, QMRA was found to be a reliable promising method for monitoring post-stenting flow changes. It should be noted that turbulence just distal to the stenosis or stent may lead to artifacts causing measurement error. [71]

Conclusion

Diagnostic vascular neurology has made amazing advances in recent decades. Various studies have shown that different modalities are complimentary in the diagnosis of vascular pathology. The development in new investigational tools offers a variety of options for the clinician to choose from, based on each method's costs and limitations and advantages, and patient risks and preferences. This evolution will continue to minimize risks and increase reliability in pathology detection and ultimately better management planning of neurovascular diseases where early detection and prompt management can affect the outcome dramatically.

References

[1] Fifi JT, Meyers PM, Lavine SD, et al., Complications of modern diagnostic cerebral angiography in an academic medical center, *J Vasc Interv Radiol,*009;20(4):442–7.

[2] Aralasmak A, Akyuz M, Ozkaynak C, Sindel T, Tuncer R (2009) CT angiography and perfusion imaging in patients with subarachnoid hemorrhage: correlation of vasospasm to perfusion abnormality. *Neuroradiology* 51:85–93.

[3] Cho YD, Park JC, Kwon BJ, Hee HM (2010) Endovascular treatment of largely thrombosed saccular aneurysms: follow-up results in ten patients. *Neuroradiology* 52:751–758.

[4] Agid R, Willinsky RA, Lee SK, terBrugge KG, Farb RI (2008) Characterization of aneurysm remnants after endovascular treatment: contrast-enhanced MR angiography versus catheter digital subtraction angiography. *AJNR Am J Neuroradiol* 29:1570–1574.

[5] Uysal E, Oztora F, Ozel A, Erturk SM, Yildirim H, Basak M (2008) Detection and evaluation of intracranial aneurysms with 16-row multislice CT angiography: comparison with conventional angiography. *Emerg Radiol* 15:311–6.

[6] Willems PW, Taeshineetanakul P, Schenk B, Brouwer PA, Terbrugge KG, Krings T. The use of 4D-CTA in the diagnostic work-up of brain arteriovenous malformations. *Neuroradiology.* 2011 Apr 5.

[7] Satoh T, Onoda K, Tsuchimoto S. Intraoperative evaluation of aneurysmal architecture: comparative study with transluminal images of 3D MR and CT angiograms. *AJNR Am J Neuroradiol.* 2003 Nov-Dec;24(10):1975-81.

[8] Inoue S, Hosoda K, Fujita A, Ohno Y, Fujii M, Kohmura E. Diagnostic imaging of cerebrovascular disease on multi-detector row computed tomography (MDCT). *Brain Nerve.* 2011 Sep;63(9):923-32.

[9] Michael Chen, MD. Interventional Neurology—Recent Advances and New Applications. *US Neurology,* 2011;7(1):37–40.

[10] Moniz E. L'encephalographie arterielle, son importance dans la localisation des tumeurs cerebrales.

[11] Tondreau, R. (1985) Egas Moniz 1874-1955. *Radiographics,* 5(6):994-997.

[12] Moniz E, *Diagnostic des tumeurs cerebrals et epreuve de l'encephalographie artérielle,* Paris: Masson, 1931.

[13] Martin NA, Bentson J, Vinuela F, et al. Intraoperative digital subtraction angiography and the surgical treatment of intracranial aneurysms and vascular malformations. *J Neurosurg* 1990;73:526–533

[14] Alexander TD, Macdonald RL, Wier B, Kowalczuk A. Intraoperative angiography in cerebral aneurysm surgery: a prospective study of 100 craniotomies. *Neurosurgery* 1996;19:10–16.

[15] Timothy J. Kaufmann, David F. Kallmes, *Diagnostic Cerebral Angiography: Archaic and Complication-Prone or Here to Stay for Another 80 Years?,* AJR:190, June 2008.

[16] Andersson M, Carstensen B, Visfeldt J. Leukemia and other related hematological disorders among Danish patients exposed to Thorotrast. *Radiat Res* 1993; 134:224–233.

[17] Thiex R, Norbash AM, Frerichs KU. The safety of dedicated-team catheter-based diagnostic cerebral angiography in the era of advanced noninvasive imaging. *AJNR Am J Neuroradiol.* 2010 Feb;31(2):230-4. Epub 2009 Sep 24.

[18] Hoh BL, Cheung AC, Rabinov JD, Pryor JC, Carter BS, Ogilvy CS. Results of a prospective protocol of computed tomographic angiography in place of catheter angiography as the only diagnostic and pretreatment planning study for cerebral aneurysms by a combined neurovascular team. *Neurosurgery* 2004; 54:1329–1340.

[19] Khashayar Farsad, Alexander C. Mamourian, Clifford J. Eskey and Jonathan A. Friedman Computed Tomographic Angiography as an Adjunct to Digital Subtraction Angiography for the Pre-Operative Assessment of Cerebral Aneurysms. *The Open Neurology Journal,* 2009, 3, 1-7 1.

[20] Anderson GB, Steinke DE, Petruk KC, Ashforth R, Findlay JM. Computed tomographic angiography versus digital subtraction angiography for the diagnosis and early treatment of ruptured intracranial aneurysms. *Neurosurgery* 1999;45:1315–1320.

[21] McKinney AM, Truwit CL, Palmer CS, Teksam M. Intracranial aneurysms: is the diagnostic accuracy rate of multidetector CT angiography equivalent to that of three-dimensional rotational conventional angiography? *Radiology.* 2008 Mar;246(3):982; author reply 982-3.

[22] Teran W. Colen, Lilian C. Wang, Basavaraj V. Ghodke, Wendy A. Cohen, William Hollingworth, Yoshimi Anzai. *Effectiveness of MDCT Angiography for the Detection of Intracranial Aneurysms in Patients with Nontraumatic Subarachnoid Hemorrhage.* AJR:189, October 2007.

[23] Abe T, Hirohata M, Tanaka N, Uchiyama Y, Kojima K, Fujimoto K, Norbash AM, Hayabuchi N. Clinical benefits of rotational 3D angiography in endovascular treatment of ruptured cerebral aneurysm. *AJNR Am J Neuroradiol.* 2002 Apr;23(4):686-8.

[24] Nishimura S, Hirai T, Shigematsu Y, Kitajima M, Morioka M, Kai Y, Minoda R, Uetani H, Murakami R, Yamashita Y. Evaluation of Brain and Head and Neck Tumors with 4D Contrast-Enhanced MR Angiography at 3T. *AJNR Am J Neuroradiol.* 2011 Nov 24.

[25] Gailloud P, Oishi S, Carpenter J, Murphy KJ. Three-dimensional digital angiography: new tool for simultaneous three-dimensional rendering of vascular and osseous information during rotational angiography. *AJNR Am J Neuroradiol.* 2004 Apr;25(4):571-3.

[26] Hochmuth A, Spetzger U, Schumacher M. Comparison of three-dimensional rotational angiography with digital subtraction angiography in the assessment of ruptured cerebral aneurysms. *AJNR Am J Neuroradiol* 2002;23:1199–1205.

[27] Hirai T, Korogi Y, Suginohara K, et al. Clinical usefulness of unsubtracted 3D digital angiography compared with rotational digital angiography in the pretreatment evaluation of intracranial aneurysms. *AJNR Am J Neuroradiol* 2003;24:1067–1074.

[28] Sugahara T, Korogi Y, Nakashima K, Hamatake S, Honda S, Takahashi M. Comparison of 2D and 3D digital subtraction angiography in evaluation of intracranial aneurysms. *AJNR Am J Neuroradiol* 2002;23:1545–1552.

[29] Piotin M, Gailloud P, Bidaut L, et al. CT angiography, MR angiography and rotational digital subtraction angiography for volumetric assessment of intracranial aneurysms: an experimental study. *Neuroradiology* 2003;45:404–409.

[30] Chappell ET, Moure FC, Good MC. Comparison of computed tomographic angiography with digital subtraction angiography in the diagnosis of cerebral aneurysms: a meta-analysis. *Neurosurgery* 2003;52:624–631, discussion630–621.

[31] Hirai T, Korogi Y, Ono K, et al. Preoperative evaluation of intracranial aneurysms: usefulness of intraarterial 3D CT angiography and conventional angiography with a combined unit—initial experience. *Radiology* 2001;220:499–505.

[32] Nishihara M, Tamaki N. Usefulness of volume-rendered three-dimensional computed tomographic angiography for surgical planning in treating unruptured paraclinoid internal carotid artery aneurysms. *Kobe J Med Sci* 2001;47:221–230.

[33] Gailloud P, Oishi S, Murphy K. Three-dimensional fusion digital subtraction angiography: new reconstruction algorithm for simultaneous three-dimensional rendering of osseous and vascular information obtained during rotational angiography. *AJNR Am J Neuroradiol.* 2005 Apr;26(4):908-11.

[34] Benndorf G. Color-coded digital subtraction angiography: the end of a monochromatic era? *AJNR Am J Neuroradiol.* 2010 May;31(5):925-7. Epub 2010 Apr 15.

[35] Hunter GJ, Hunter JV, Brown NJ. Parametric imaging using digital subtraction angiography. *Br J Radiol* 1986;59:7–11.

[36] Hunter JV. Parametric imaging applied to renal digital subtraction angiography: establishment of normal ranges. *Urol Radiol* 1986; 8: 204– 08.

[37] Wintermark M, Lev MH. FDA investigates the safety of brain perfusion CT. AJNR *Am J Neuroradiol* 2010;31:2–3. Epub 2009 Nov 5.

[38] Strother CM, Bender F, Deuerling-Zheng Y, Royalty K, Pulfer KA, Baumgart J, Zellerhoff M, Aagaard-Kienitz B, Niemann DB, Lindstrom ML. Parametric color

coding of digital subtraction angiography. *AJNR Am J Neuroradiol.* 2010 May;31(5):919-24. Epub 2010 Feb 18.

[39] Hashimoto H, Iida J, Hironaka Y, Okada M, Sakaki T. Use of spiral computerized tomography angiography in patients with subarachnoid hemorrhage in whom subtraction angiography did not reveal cerebral aneurysms. J Neurosurg 2000;92:278–283.

[40] Amagasaki K, Sato T, Kakizawa T, Shimizu T. Treatment of ruptured anterior circulation aneurysm based on computerized tomography angiography: surgical results and indications for additional digital subtraction angiography. J Clin Neurosci 2002;9 : 22–29.

[41] Boet R, Poon WS, Lam JM, Yu SC. The surgical treatment of intracranial aneurysms based on computer tomographic angiography alone: streamlining the acute management of symptomatic aneurysms. Acta Neurochir (Wien) 2003; 145:101 –105; discussion, 105.

[42] Villablanca JP, Jahan R, Hooshi P, et al. Detection and characterization of very small cerebral aneurysms by using 2D and 3D helical CT angiography. AJNR 2002;23 :1187 –1198.

[43] Bash S, Villablanca JP, Jahan R, Duckwiler G, Tillis M, Kidwell C, Saver J, Sayre J. Intracranial vascular stenosis and occlusive disease: evaluation with CT angiography, MR angiography, and digital subtraction angiography. AJNR Am J Neuroradiol. 2005 May;26(5):1012-21.

[44] Chen Y, Manness W, Kattner K. Application of CT angiography of complex cerebrovascular lesions during surgical decision making. Skull Base. 2004 Nov;14(4):185-93; discussion 193.

[45] Tomura N, Otani T, Sakuma I, Takahashi S, Nishii T, Watarai J. Three-dimensional bone-free computed tomographic angiography of aneurysms near the skull base using a new bone-removal application. Jpn J Radiol. 2009 Jan;27(1):31-6. Epub 2009 Feb 8.

[46] Zhang LJ, Wu SY, Niu JB, Zhang ZL, Wang HZ, Zhao YE, Chai X, Zhou CS, Lu GM. Dual-energy CT angiography in the evaluation of intracranial aneurysms: image quality, radiation dose, and comparison with 3D rotational digital subtraction angiography. AJR Am J Roentgenol. 2010 Jan;194(1):23-30.

[47] Klingebiel R, Siebert E, Diekmann S, Wiener E, Masuhr F, Wagner M, Bauknecht HC, Dewey M, Bohner G (2009) 4-D Imaging in cerebrovascular disorders by using 320-slice CT: feasibility and preliminary clinical experience. Acad Radiol 16:123–129.

[48] Brouwer PA, Bosman T, van Walderveen MA, Krings T, Leroux AA, Willems PW (2010) Dynamic 320-section CT angiography in cranial arteriovenous shunting lesions. AJNR Am J Neuroradiol 31:767–770.

[49] Cademartiri F, Mollet N, van der Lugt A, et al. Non-invasive 16-row multislice CT coronary angiography: usefulness of saline chaser. *Eur Radiol* 2004;14 : 178–183.

[50] Flohr T, Stierstorfer K, Bruder H, Simon J, Schaller S. New technical developments in multislice CT. Part 1. Approaching isotropic resolution with sub-millimeter 16-slice scanning. *Rofo*2002 ; 174:839 –845.

[51] Kato Y, Nair S, Sano H, Sanjaykumar MS, Katada K, Hayakawa M, Kanno T. Multi-slice 3D-CTA - an improvement over single slice helical CTA for cerebral aneurysms. *Acta Neurochir (Wien).* 2002 Jul;144(7):715-22.

[52] Haage P, Schmitz-Rode T, Hubner D, Piroth W, Gunther RW. Reduction of contrast material dose and artifacts by a saline flush using a double power injector in helical CT of the thorax. *AJR*2000 ; 174:1049 –1053.

[53] Hopper KD, Mosher TJ, Kasales CJ, TenHave TR, Tully DA, Weaver JS. Thoracic spiral CT: delivery of contrast material pushed with injectable saline solution in a power injector. *Radiology* 1997 ; 205:269 –271.

[54] Tamura Y, Utsunomiya D, Sakamoto T, Hirai T, Nishiharu T, Urata J, Yamashita Y.. Reduction of contrast material volume in 3D angiography of the brain using MDCT. *AJR Am J Roentgenol.* 2010 Aug;195(2):455-8.

[55] Marckmann P., Skov L., Rossen K., et al: Nephrogenic systemic fibrosis: suspected causative role of gadodiamide used for contrast-enhanced magnetic resonance imaging. *J Am Soc Nephrol* 17. (9): 2359-2362.2006.

[56] Grobner T.: Gadolinium—a specific trigger for the development of nephrogenic fibrosing dermopathy and nephrogenic systemic fibrosis?. *Nephrol Dial* 21. (4): 1104-1108.2006.

[57] Kapsalaki EZ, Rountas CD, Fountas KN. The Role of 3 Tesla MRA in the Detection of Intracranial Aneurysms. *Int J Vasc Med.* 2012;2012:792834. Epub 2012 Jan 16.

[58] Schaafsma JD, Velthuis BK, Majoie CB, van den Berg R, Brouwer PA, Barkhof F, et al. Intracranial aneurysms treated with coil placement: test characteristics of follow-up MR angiography--multicenter study. *Radiology.* 2010;256:209–218.

[59] Wall A, Kugel H, Bachman R, Matuszewski L, Kramer S, Heindel W, et al. 3.0 T vs. 1.5 T MR angiography: in vitro comparison of intravascular stent artifacts. *J Magn Reson Imaging.* 2005;22:772–779.

[60] Wang Y, Truong TN, Yen C, Bilecen D, Watts R, Trost DW, et al. Quantitative evaluation of susceptibility and shielding effects of nitinol, platinum, cobalt-alloy, and stainless steel stents. *Magn Reson Med.* 2003;49:972–976.

[61] Takayama K, Taoka T, Nakagawa H, Myouchin K, Wada T, Sakamoto M, Fukusumi A, Iwasaki S, Kurokawa S, Kichikawa K. Usefulness of contrast-enhanced magnetic resonance angiography for follow-up of coil embolization with the enterprise stent for cerebral aneurysms. *J Comput Assist Tomogr.* 2011 Sep-Oct;35(5):568-72.

[62] Pierot L, Delcourt C, Bouquigny F, et al. Follow-up of intracranial aneurysms selectively treated with coils: prospective evaluation of contrast-enhanced MR angiography. *AJNR Am J Neuroradiol.* 2006;27:744-749.

[63] Choi JW, Roh HG, Moon WJ, Kim NR, Moon SG, Kang CH, Chun YI, Kang HS. Time-resolved 3D contrast-enhanced MRA on 3.0T: a non-invasive follow-up technique after stent-assisted coil embolization of the intracranial aneurysm. *Korean J Radiol.* 2011 Nov;12(6):662-70. Epub 2011 Sep 27.

[64] Cashen TA, Carr JC, Shin W, Walker MT, Futterer SF, Shaibani A, et al. Intracranial time-resolved contrast-enhanced MR angiography at 3T. *AJNR Am J Neuroradiol.* 2006;27:822–829.

[65] Farb RI, Agid R, Willinsky RA, Johnstone DM, Terbrugge KG. Cranial dural arteriovenous fistula: diagnosis and classification with time-resolved MR angiography at 3T. *AJNR Am J Neuroradiol.* 2009;30:1546–1551.

[66] Hadizadeh DR, Kukuk GM, Steck DT, Gieseke J, Urbach H, Tschampa HJ, Greschus S, Kovàcs A, Möhlenbruch M, Bostroem A, Schild HH, Willinek WA. AJNR Am J Neuroradiol. Noninvasive Evaluation of Cerebral Arteriovenous Malformations by 4D-

MRA for Preoperative Planning and Postoperative Follow-Up in 56 Patients: *Comparison with DSA and Intraoperative Findings.* 2012 Feb 2.

[67] Lim HK, Choi CG, Kim SM, Kim JL, Lee DH, Kim SJ, Suh DC. Detection of residual brain arteriovenous malformations after radiosurgery: diagnostic accuracy of contrast-enhanced four-dimensional MR angiography at 3.0 *T. Br J Radiol.* 2012 Jan 31.

[68] Prabhakaran S, Warrior L, Wells KR, Jhaveri MD, Chen M, Lopes DK. The utility of quantitative magnetic resonance angiography in the assessment of intracranial in-stent stenosis. *Stroke.* 2009 Mar;40(3):991-3. Epub 2009 Jan 22.

[69] Zhao M, Amin-Hanjani S, Ruland S, Curcio AP, Ostergren L, Charbel FT. Regional cerebral blood flow using quantitative MR angiography. *AJNR Am J Neuroradiol.* 2007; 28: 1470–1473.

[70] Amin-Hanjani S, Alaraj A, Calderon-Arnulphi M, Aletich VA, Thulborn KR, Charbel FT. Detection of intracranial in-stent restenosis using quantitative magnetic resonance angiography. *Stroke.* 2010 Nov;41(11):2534-8. Epub 2010 Oct 7.

[71] Prabhakaran S, Wells KR, Jhaveri MD, Lopes DK. Hemodynamic changes following wingspan stent placement--a quantitative magnetic resonance angiography study. *J Neuroimaging.* 2011 Apr;21(2):e109-13. doi: 10.1111/j.1552-6569.2009.00425.x.

In: New Developments in Angiography Research
Editors: K. I. Sanders and A. M. Jackson

ISBN: 978-1-62081-492-5

Chapter V

HEADACHE AND ENDOVASCULAR MANIPULATION

***Raquel Gil-Gouveia*[1,2] *and Isabel Pavão Martins*[1]**
[1]Department of Clinical Neurosciences (UNIC), Instituto de Medicina Molecular (IMM), Lisbon Faculty of Medicine, Lisboa, Portugal
[2]Headache Outpatient Clinic, Hospital da Luz, Lisboa, Portugal

Introduction: Although many primary headaches are attributed to structural and functional changes of intracranial vessels, studies on pain from direct stimulation of the arterial or venous walls are scarce. Intracranial endovascular procedures can be viewed as models to study that type of pain. On the other hand, the occurrence of headaches during and after endovascular procedures can be a red flag for an intracranial complication or simply a consequence of vessel manipulation.

Purpose: In this chapter we review the data about headaches related to angiography and endovascular procedures and try to correlate their mechanisms and localization. We also attempt to characterize clinically these headaches, in order to identify relevant clinical alarm signs for evaluation of headaches related to endovascular procedures.

Methods: A review of publications in English, French or Portuguese language with the key words vascular headache, headache, migraine, angiography, embolization, endovascular interventions was sought. Primary headaches were excluded.

Results: Headache occurs frequently (19 to 65%) during angiography and endovascular procedures, always in consequence of a specific manoeuvre and it is sharp, intense, brief without accompanying symptoms. It projects to the scalp area in the distribution of the nocipetive innervation of the involved artery. Headache frequently (33 to 47%) appears in the 24 hours after angiography and it is usually self-limited, mild and uncharacteristic. Angiography and endovascular procedures do not increase the likelihood of future recurrent headaches.

INTRODUCTION

Cerebral angiography, introduced by Egas Moniz in 1927 [1] was the first imaging procedure of the intracranial structures and has been since an important diagnostic tool for intracranial disorders. Soon after its first use in diagnosis, it was applied for therapeutic purposes for a carotid-cavernous fistula, in 1932[2] Despite the major developments in other brain imaging methods that took place in the last 3 decades, and allowed unique anatomical detail and functional studies without the use of ionizing radiation, modern angiography is still the gold standard for the diagnosis of intracranial vascular disorders [3-5]. Its therapeutic application was much improved by technological developments and today intervention neurorradiology is used routinely world-wide.

Headache is one of the cerebrovascular symptoms that lead to the performance of an angiography or endovascular procedure. In addition, headaches can also happen during and after angiography and other endovascular procedures, and can be entirely benign as a consequence of the procedure *per se* or a warning sign of intracranial complications of the baseline disorder or procedure. Yet, little information is available to help clinicians identify threatening headaches or to predict and prevent the discomfort associated with the most benign headache complaints.

Further to that, on theoretical grounds, angiography and endovascular procedures can be viewed as models to study vascular headache in real time, i.e., headache due to direct endovascular stimulation, a knowledge that can be extrapolated to better understand the headaches of vascular disorders and vascular changes occurring during primary headaches.

We will start by briefly reviewing the anatomy and neurochemistry of the intracranial nociception and the clinical correlation of headache to intracranial vascular disorders. We will then present a systematic review of the literature with the key words vascular headache, headache, migraine, angiography, embolization and endovascular interventions in order to characterize particular patterns of pain associated to embolization and angiography.

1. Intracranial Nociception

Despite the evolutive importance of intracranial contents, only three intracranial structures are pain-sensitive – the meninges, the vessels and the nerves.

In the main intracranial arteries, nerve bundles are located in the periadventitial tissue, surrounded by a perineurim and contain both myelinated and unmyelinated fibbers. The number of periadventicial nerve fibbers increases in proportion to the calibre of the vessel and when arteries reach the size of an arteriole, only unmyelinated fibbers persist [6]. Arteries penetrating the pia mater into the brain become surrounded by a perivascular sheath, and loose their adventitial layer and most of its innervation [6]. In result, intraparenchymal vessels have sparse innervation contrasting with the major extraparenchymal trunks that are richly innervated, such as the internal carotid, the anterior, middle and posterior cerebral arteries, basilar trunk, vertebral (bilateral innervation is only present in 2/3 of individuals) and, sporadically, the proximal portions of the posterior inferior and anterior superior cerebellar arteries [7].

Nerve fibbers in the dural tissue originate from Ruffini-like terminals (that act as mechanoreceptors) and encapsulated and lamellated terminals (that detect volume changes). The leptomeningeal nerve terminals additionally contain chemoreceptors [8]. Meningeal vessels have an extensive innervation, containing the same type of receptors [8]. Vascularisation of the intracranial meninges is composed of large dural arteries, dural venous sinuses in the periostal layer and of a dense capillary network in the meningeal layer, adjacent to the arachnoid [8]

Nociceptive innervation of the intracranial arteries and meninges is supplied by branches of the trigeminal nerve. Its terminals are rich in glutamate and calcitonine gene related peptide (CGRP) [9] that mediate nociception, but also substance P (SP) and Neurokinin A (NKA) [10] that mediate arterial relaxation.

Autonomic innervation of intracranial arteries is located in the adventitial-medial border [11]. Sympathetic innervation is more abundant in cortical vessels while small arteries and arterioles are innervated by single fibbers only [10]. The dura also contains catecholaminergic nerve fibers that are most abundant in the perivascular dural zone and in the basal region [12-14]. Sympathetic aminergic fibbers are also found, in abundance, under the endothelium of the dural sinuses, and its number decreases progressively in deep cerebral and superficial veins [15] suggesting the ability of venoconstriction. Most sympathetic fibbers derive from the superior cervical ganglion [16] and contain Neuropeptide-Y (NPY) and noradrenaline (NA), both potent vasoconstrictors [10].

Parasympathetic innervation arises from the sphenopalatine, otic and small local ganglia at the base of the skull [16], that supply arteries and cranial dura [14] with a sparse network of cholinergic and Vasointestinal Peptide (VIP) containing fibbers, acting as potent vasodilators [10]. Cerebral veins have peptidergic neurons containing VIP and SP that may also influence venous diameter [15], yet no cholinergic fibbers have been documented in the venous system.

Sensory innervation of the intracranial compartment follows a somatotopic organization, as nociception of the intracranial compartment is divided in two territories – fibbers supplying the spinal and posterior cranial fossa dura mater arise from the first three cervical posterior nerve roots (C2,C3) while the supratentorial portion of the dura mater, the major arterial trunks of the Circle of Willis and the middle meningeal and pial arteries are supplied by afferents of the trigeminal nerve, specially the first division [8, 17, 18]. Irrespective of their nerve trajectory, all nociceptive fibbers arising in the intracranial compartment project to the same central nucleus – the pars caudalis of the spinal trigeminal nucleus (trigeminal nucleus caudalis, TNC), that extends from the lower pons to the third cervical segment of the spinal cord [17].

The somatotopic innervation of the dura implies that mechanical, electrical and thermal stimulation of the intracranial dura in different locations gives origin to head pain localized to specific areas of the head [13, 19]. However, the pattern of pain referral is not consistent, as some dural areas are more sensitive (ex. perivascular dura) and there is a significant overlap between different territories (13). In addition, convergence of meningeal and facial afferent inputs onto central trigeminal neurons may result in facilitation and referred pain patterns [20].

The pain originating by arterial and venous intracranial stimulation is not as clearly referred to specific locations. Stimulation of the human middle meningeal artery (by clamping or endothermy) has inconsistently produced homolateral acute sharp pain in the temple or above the ear[21]. Displacement or pressure on the human internal carotid artery may result in homolateral pain in the eye or temple [21]. Stimulation of the vertebral and basilar arteries may origin pain in the back of the head and in the neck [22]. There are also inconsistent observations of pain produced by electrical stimulation of the human superior sagital sinus, which sometimes produces pain in the homolateral vertex, forehead, eye or temple [21]. Cortical veins and arteries and the choroid plexus were never documented as pain sensitive structures [15].

2. Clinical Contribute: Naturally Occurrig Headache in Intracranial Vascular Disorders

Despite the inconsistency of these observations, vasodilatation of intracranial blood vessels was thought to be the underlying mechanism for migraine headache for many years [23]. Still today debate exists about the contribution of dilatation of extra- and intracerebral arteries in the pathophysiology of migraine [24, 25].

Several intracranial vascular disorders have very consistent high rates of headache at presentation, such as cerebral venous thrombosis (89%) [26], subarachnoid haemorrhage (74%) [27] and hemorrhagic stroke (30 to 60%) [28]. In these conditions, the headaches' origin might not relate to damage to the vessel itself but rather be due to increased intracranial pressure and/or direct or indirect meningeal stimulation [28, 29].

Other vascular disorders can also present with headache that is hardly related to these mechanisms. As an example, carotid dissection presents with ipsilateral anterior headache or facial pain in 78% of patients on average 9 days before the onset of ischemic brain lesions [30]. Sixty-nine percent of vertebral dissection patients present with ipsilateral or bilateral occipital headache or neck pain on average 3 days before additional symptoms arise [30]. These headaches are thought to originate from direct vessel damage, as the tear in the intimal lining allows the formation of intramural hematoma damaging periadventitial nociceptive and sympathetic fibbers [29] producing pain with a location suggestive of the nociceptive innervation pattern [8, 17, 18].

Intracranial morphologically intact arteries can also produce thunderclap or acute severe isolated headaches, as occurs in the reversible cerebral vasoconstriction syndrome on average a week before other symptoms arise [31, 32]. Its origin is probably a transient disturbance in the control of cerebral vascular tone, either spontaneous or secondary, producing reversible severe diffuse, multifocal, segmental vasospasm of the large and medium-sized arteries in the anterior and posterior circulation, that theoretically disturb pain sensitive fibbers in vessel walls [31].

Headache occurring during ischemic stroke, lacunar infarts or TIA has probably a very different aetiology and pathophysiology [33, 34] and will not be discussed further in this review.

3. Headache and Angiography or Endovascular Procedures

Taking into account their rich innervations, as explained above, headaches might be expected to occur during and after cerebral angiography and endovascular procedures independently of any vascular or parenchyma damage. Furthermore, those procedures provide good experimental human models to the study headaches evoked by intra-luminal stimulation of intracranial arteries. We aimed to review the existing data about headache evoked by endovascular procedures, in order to characterize the benign headaches that might occur during or after arterial manipulation performed in these procedures.

We searched Pub Med with the terms "vascular headache", "headache and angiography", "headache and endovascular intervention/ procedure", "headache and embolization", "migraine and angiography", "migraine and endovascular procedures/ intervention" and "migraine and embolization". When more than one thousand references were obtained, the search was limited to "Clinical Trial or Meta-Analysis or Practice Guideline or Randomized Controlled Trial or Review". We also identified relevant published work by searching the reference list of articles retrieved from this search. Historical references were added to the list obtained electronically. Relevant reports published in English, French or Portuguese were reviewed. The final reference list was generated on the basis of relevance to the aim of this review.

Headache is often not reported in meta-analysis and large prospective studies about complications of cerebral angiography [35-37], although it was described at least since 1964 [38]. A retrospective analysis of 19826 procedures has reported 0.8% headache occurrence within 24h of diagnostic cerebral angiography. Being a retrospective study, this data is a clearly underestimation as only clinical relevant data is usually registered – in this specific study; data from headache occurrence was missing in 7037 procedures [39]. Specific studies focusing on the occurrence of headache during or after angiography or endovascular procedures are very scarce (table 1).

Headache during Endovascular Procedures - Most of the existent data reflects the occurrence of headache during endovascular procedures [40-47] and findings are very consistent – pain is always related to a specific endovascular manoeuvre, is always sharp, moderate to intense, brief (seconds to minutes) and ipsilateral to the stimulated side. It is an isolated pain, without accompanying symptoms. Its frequency is variable, ranging from 19% [40] to 64% [47] between series, this variability probably relates to small sample sizes. Specific location of pain relates to stimulation site [40-42, 44-47], reflecting known patterns of vessel nociceptive innervations [17, 18] and probably representing a referred pain pattern.

This type of sharp brief pain has a clinical similar in thunderclap headache, that might occur as a consequence of vessel rupture in subarachnoid haemorrhage or in vasospasm such as occurring during the reversible vasoconstriction syndrome. Its onset and location patterns are highly suggestive of a cause-effect relationship to endovascular manipulation and the type of stimulus that usually results in this type of headache results of high focal pressure of the arterial wall (balloon inflation [40, 44-47], contrast [40-42] or glue injection [40]) or to focal mechanical distension, although there is little angiographic evidence arterial calibre changes during these manoeuvres [47]. In carotid pain, a relation was found with the incidence of intimal flaps, reflecting a relation to the stretching of the vessel during angioplasty, yet no correlation was found to the extent of vessel dilatation [47]. Although appealing, the mechanistic explanation might not be the correct one. Chemical effects of contrast agents [41, 42, 48] on the endothelial wall may also play a role, by themselves or in addition to increase in local pressure. A relation with contrast volume rather than its iodine concentration may argue in favour of the mechanical distension [40].

Risk factors for the occurrence of headache during endovascular procedures were only documented in two studies [40, 47]. Headache occurred with higher frequency in embolizations [40], when compared to diagnostic angiography and during carotid angioplasties with intraprocedural bradicardia [47] (reinforcing a possible role for mechanical stimulation), in females and in patients with frequent previous headaches [40] and in patients with history of myocardial infarction [47], suggesting that host and vessel susceptibility factors also have influence. These headaches are mostly benign, very brief, resolve spontaneously, and are not associated with concomitant neurological symptoms or signs.

Table 1. Studies on Headache and Endovascular Procedures

Author, Year	Study Description	Sample size	Main Findings
Hauge, 1954(41)	Prospective observation of headache and focal symptoms during vertebral angiography	Patients 76 Procedures 90	Vertebral characterization and contrast (diotrast) injection produced mostly contralateral visual phenomena suggestive of aura + ipsilateral frontal headache (48/90) + facial pain, tearing, tinnitus + nausea and vomiting + diffuse headache (at a later stage).
Hauge, 1986(42)	Prospective observation of headache and focal symptoms during and after vertebral angiography	Patients 56 Procedures 56	Vertebral characterization and contrast (less toxic) injection produced immediate ipsilateral cervico-occipital pain, facial pain, tearing, rinorrhea + nausea and vomiting (10-15 min) + visual aura symptoms + bulbar symptoms. After 1h 50% patients had frontal bilateral headache (lasting 7 to 72h) + nausea, vomiting, hallucinations, perception disorders, amnesia and bulbar symptoms.
Shuaib, 1988(43)	Retrospective review of migraine patients during and within 24h of cerebral angiography	Patients 142 Procedures 149	Typical migraine headache occurred in 3 patients
Nichols, 1990(44)	Prospective observation of headache during embolization therapy for AVM, with balloon occlusion of the ICA and MCA	Patients 18 Procedures 26	11/18 focal brief ipsilateral headache during balloon inflation: - on the cantus during ICA stimulation - retro-orbital during middle MCA stimulation - above the eye during distal MCA stimulation
Nichols, 1993(46)	Prospective observation of headache during embolization therapy for AVM, with balloon occlusion of the vertebral and basilar	Patients 1 Procedures 1	Focal brief ipsilateral headache during balloon inflation: - on the neck and shoulder during proximal vertebral stimulation - ear, mastoid and neck during middle proximal vertebral stimulation + forehead and cheek during proximal vertebral artery stimulation - skull vertex, occiput and neck during proximal basilar stimulation
Martins, 1993(45)	Prospective observation of headache during embolization therapy for AVM and aneurysms	Patients 11 Procedures 11 Pedicules occluded 38	22/ 38 episodes of sudden onset intense (excruciating in 7/22) pain lasting less that 10 min (in 20/22) and with gradual disappearance, 1/22 had nausea, 0/22 had aura, 1/22 had transient focal deficit always ipsilateral to the stimulated artery. Location of pain was dependent of the stimulated artery but was always on trigeminal territory.
Munari, 1994(47)	Review of carotid artery stenoses treated by transluminal angioplasty	Patients 42 Procedures 42	27/42 ipsilateral sharp moderate (16/27) neck pain with balloon inflation lasting a few seconds to several minutes (7/27) up to 3h (3/27), pattern of pain radiation was related to the stimulated segment of ICA; its occurrence was related to risk factors
Ramadan, 1995(52)	Prospective standardized observation of headache after angiography	Patients 45 Procedures 45	15/45 had post-angiography headache that developed after 2h unilateral (9/15) and throbbing (6/15), mostly without other symptoms. 8/15 had previous headaches (5 TTH, 3 Migraine) versus 7/30 of the non headache group. No other risk factors identified.

Author, Year	Study Description	Sample size	Main Findings
Beekmanm 2001(53)	3 case reports of migraine developing after routine angiography and embolization of AVM	Patients 3 Procedures 3	Patient 1 - 1st episode of migraine with visual aura on the right hemifield, with left sided migraine-like headache developing 1h after embolization of the left sided occipital and maxillary arteries (for AVM treatment), lasting < 24h Patient 2 – Hours after routine control angiography (left ICA embolized aneurysm) developed visual, sensitive and hemiplegic aura for 2h with typical migraine-like headache lasting < 24h Patient 3 – Two hours after glue embolization of left occipital AVM had right sided hemianopia (was left with quadrantanopia) and severe migraine-like headache that lasted a week
Gil-Gouveia, 2007(40)	Prospective standardized observation of headache during angiography and endovascular procedures	Patients 107 Procedures 122 Evaluated procedures 68	13/68 had stabbing (5/13) or pressure-like (4/13) mild or moderate (6/13) unilateral (8/13) short-lasting pain, (2 to 30 seconds) always triggered by a specific homolateral (in all but 1 case) maneuver: injection of contrast (9/13) or cyanoacrylate (2/13) or filling a balloon (2/13). Female gender and frequent previous headaches were risk factors.
Gil-Gouveia, 2008(50)	Prospective standardized observation of headache after angiography and endovascular procedures	Patients 107 Procedures 122	35% had mild stabbing bilateral headaches starting following an headache free period after angiography; risk factor: female gender 49% had recurrent headaches 6 months after the procedure, risk factor: previous headache
Takigawa, 2011(51)	Retrospective database review of headache and fever after aneurism embolization comparing bare with bioactive coils	Patients 88 Procedures 92	47% had mild headache after embolization, bioactive coils more often than bare coils (66% versus 25%) and headaches lasted longer (3,4 versus 2,3 days).

If happening during carotid angioplasty they don't increase the risk of brain ischemia following the procedure [47] and if happening during intracranial angiography and endovascular procedures there is also no increased risk of intraprocedural, early (<24h) or late (~ 6 months) neurological complications [49].

Headache after Endovascular Procedures – Data on headache occurrence after endovascular procedures is even scarcer. Clinically, it is difficult to identify these headaches as, nowadays, patients are sedated during those procedures and many patients undergoing endovascular procedures or angiography have baseline disorders that do manifest with headaches, such as subarachnoid haemorrhage, that of course is a risk factor for immediate post-angiography headache occurrence [50].

Early (<24h) post-angiography headaches are probably the only headaches listed in some studies dealing with complications of angiography and endovascular procedures [35-37, 39]. There are three studies analysing early (< 24h) post-angiography or post-procedure headaches [50-52] and two report a delay of a few hours on headache onset, after the procedure, with the development of a mild to moderate self-limited isolated headache, without consistent characteristics [50, 52]. This delayed onset had been described previously [43, 53] and it was speculated that its occurrence might be due to a trigger effect of the procedure itself, either by acting as a stressor or by inducing chemical or inflammatory changes within the vessel [50-52].

Female gender was a risk factor for the development of early post-angiography headaches in one study [50] and the occurrence of previous headache in other [52], suggesting a baseline susceptibility status. The use of bioactive coils was also associated with a higher risk of post-procedure headache occurrence [51], probably due to the higher occurrence of intra-aneurismal inflammatory changes.

The mild, unspecific an non-progressive nature of these headaches is quite reassuring as they are easily distinguished from acute or progressive headaches that might herald intracranial complications after the procedure, either due to the procedure itself or to the baseline disorder. Nevertheless, its frequency is high – from 33% to 46.6% [50-52] - so it should be listed as an expected occurrence after such procedures and symptomatic medication should be offered to patients, if needed.

A few case reports describe the development of post-angiography attacks of migraine with aura [53-55], yet in five of the described cases vessel calibre changes were documented during the symptoms. It is possible that arterial stimulation induced the cortical spreading depression in these patients but it is also possible that focal neurological symptoms were a consequence of localized blood flow changes, due to vasospasm. Transient focal signs of the earlier reports were later related to toxicity of the contrast media [42] and in more recent reports reversibility was, sometimes, incomplete [53], suggesting that these episodes could be, in fact, due ischemic insult. In any case, none of the systematic observational studies [50-52] identified further occurrence of migraine with aura after angiography, suggesting its anecdotal association with the procedure.

Some patients complain about the occurrence of recurrent headaches after angiography or endovascular procedures. The one study designed to evaluate these headaches (at 6 months) reported almost 50% of headache incidence. One fifth of patients did relate the onset of their complaints with the procedure, although the only risk factor indentified for recurrent headache occurrence after angiography was a previous diagnosis of migraine [50]. In fact, these late recurrent headaches were generally frequent (average 20/month) self-limited short lasting (around 3h) episodes of unilateral non-throbbing mild headache with phonophobia and photophobia but with little nausea, representing typical episodes of migraine (or tension type headache) and correlated with the same previous headache diagnoses [50]. As so, angiography is not expected to resolve or improve previous headache patterns, despite some suggestive reports [56].

The late recurrent headache has probably no causal relation to the procedure. A temporal relation is reported by patients but it could relate to recall bias or increased concern about neurological symptoms, after an acute event that resulted in the diagnostic or therapeutically intervention [50]. This is important to take into account if one wants to call those headaches symptomatic.

Conclusion

The International Classification of Headache Disorders [57] includes entities such as carotid angioplasty headache (ICDH-II code 6.5.3), headache attributed to intracranial endovascular procedures (ICDH-II code 6.5.4) and angiography headache (ICDH-II code 6.5.5) yet their diagnostic criteria are too general and its description is outdated, referring only to earlier studies on angiography. After saying that, this review is a good example of the difficulties in performing systematic observational studies on large series of patients because there are too many uncontrolled variables that prevent definite conclusions. As start-off examples, practicability and ethics prevent these studies to be performed in healthy volunteers, so a very important confounder is the existence of a previous vascular disorder (of high suspicion of such) – many vascular disorders are complicated by headaches and vessel changes can increase susceptibility to headaches. Uncontrolled variables of the procedure itself also play a major role – included studies have different types of contrasts, embolic material, glues, coils and ballons [40-42, 44-47, 50-52], not to mention the large variation of volumes administered in each maneuver, the ability to document vessel distention or vasospasm, variations in intraprocedural blood pressure, anesthetic and analgesics used s, the stress of the procedures, etc. The individual characteristics of the patient are easier to systematize although the occurrence of previous headaches is always determined by history and concurrent medication or intervening illnesses might influence their ability to provide a correct history.

Nevertheless, this effort to systematize current knowledge has heralded some conclusions that must be assumed in line with the - limitations mentioned above. Headache occurring during angiography and endovascular procedures has a striking resemblance to pain originating from arterial rupture or vasospasm [27, 28, 31] with a very sudden onset, brief duration, and a location that reflects the anatomical distribution of nociceptive arterial nerve fibers [18, 19]. It occurs frequently (19% to 64% of cases [40, 47]) and is always due to a specific maneuver that implies increased intra-arterial pressure or the contact of certain substances with the vessel wall (contrast dye, glue, coils, ballons [40, 44-47]) since ithas not been described with saline injections during the procedure. Its most likely cause is vessel distention, as it occurs during embolization procedures and with higher volumes of contrast injection [40] and is associated with intraprocedural bradicardia in carotid angioplasties [47]. Non procedure-related risk factors for its occurrence are female gender, previous frequent headaches [40] and a past history of myocardial infarction [47], suggesting some influence of host and vessel susceptibility factors. Their occurrence does not increase the risk of post-procedure immediate or late recurrent headaches [50] nor of angiographic early or late complications [47, 49].

Headache occurring in the first 24 hours after angiography and endovascular procedures is also frequent (33% to 46.6% (50-52)) and often occurs with a delay of hours after the procedure. It is mild and uncharacteristic and females (50), patients with previous headaches (52), and the use of bioactive coils in embolization procedures (51) are considered risk factors for the development of headache It seems like a delayed response to local inflammatory, chemical or mechanical changes within the vessel (50-52) in susceptible individuals. Its occurrence also does not increase the risk of late recurrent headaches (50) nor of angiographic early or late complications(47, 49).

Angiography and endovascular procedures apparently do not increase the frequency of recurrent headaches persisting 6 months after the procedure, despite the fact that 20% of patients relate the onset of their symptoms with the procedure and/or the disease that justified the need for the procedure (50). Late recurrent headaches after angiography and endovascular procedures are associated with previous headaches, either migraine or tension-type headaches. Despite previous reports, migraine does not seem to act as a risk factor for neurological complications during or after angiography or endovascular procedures (50-52).

References

[1] Moniz E. Encéphalographie artérielle: son importance dans le diagnostic des tumours cérébrales. *Revue Neurologique,* 1927;1:48-72.

[2] Pool JL. The development of modern intracranial aneurysm surgery. *Neurosurgery,* 1977;1:233-237.

[3] Thaker NG, Turner JD, Cobb WS, et al. Computed tomographic angiography versus digital subtraction angiography for the postoperative detection of residual aneurysms: a single-institution series and meta-analysis. *J. Neurointerv. Surg*., 2011.

[4] Mossa-Basha M, Chen J, Gandhi D. Imaging of cerebral arteriovenous malformations and dural arteriovenous fistulas. *Neurosurg. Clin. N. Am*., 2012;23:27-42.

[5] Feldmann E, Wilterdink JL, Kosinski A, et al. The Stroke Outcomes and Neuroimaging of Intracranial Atherosclerosis (SONIA) trial. *Neurology,* 2007;68:2099-2106.

[6] Dahl E. The innervation of the cerebral arteries. *J. Anat*., 1973;115:53-63.

[7] Fang H, Birmingham A. Cerebral arterial innervations in man. *Archives of Neurology,* 1961;4:651-656.

[8] Fricke B, Andres KH, Von During M. Nerve fibers innervating the cranial and spinal meninges: morphology of nerve fiber terminals and their structural integration. *Microsc. Res. Tech*., 2001;53:96-105.

[9] Storer RJ, Akerman S, Goadsby PJ. Calcitonin gene-related peptide (CGRP) modulates nociceptive trigeminovascular transmission in the cat. *Br. J. Pharmacol*., 2004;142:1171-1181.

[10] Edvinsson L, Jansen I, Cunha e Sa M, Gulbenkian S. Demonstration of neuropeptide containing nerves and vasomotor responses to perivascular peptides in human cerebral arteries. *Cephalalgia,* 1994;14:88-96.

[11] Edvinsson L, Goadsby PJ. Neuropeptides in the cerebral circulation: relevance to headache. *Cephalalgia,* 1995;15:272-276.

[12] Cavallotti D, Artico M, De Santis S, Iannetti G, Cavallotti C. Catecholaminergic innervation of the human dura mater involved in headache. *Headache,* 1998;38:352-355.

[13] Kemp WJ, 3rd, Tubbs RS, Cohen-Gadol AA. The Innervation of the Cranial Dura Mater: Neurosurgical Case Correlates and a Review of the Literature. *World Neurosurg*., 2011.

[14] Artico M, Cavallotti C. Catecholaminergic and acetylcholine esterase containing nerves of cranial and spinal dura mater in humans and rodents. *Microsc. Res. Tech*., 2001;53:212-220.

[15] Nakakita K, Imai H, Kamei I, et al. Innervation of the cerebral veins as compared with the cerebral arteries: a histochemical and electron microscopic study. *J. Cereb. Blood Flow Metab*., 1983;3:127-132.

[16] Uddman R, Edvinsson L. Neuropeptides in the cerebral circulation. *Cerebrovasc. Brain Metab. Rev*., 1989;1:230-252.

[17] FitzGerald M, Folan-Curran J. Clinical Neuroanatomy and related neuroscience, Fourth ed. Edinburgh: W. B. Saunders, 2002.
[18] May A, Goadsby PJ. The trigeminovascular system in humans: pathophysiologic implications for primary headache syndromes of the neural influences on the cerebral circulation. *J. Cereb. Blood Flow Metab.,* 1999;19:115-127.
[19] Feindel W, Penfield W, McNaughton F. The tentorial nerves and localization of intracranial pain in man. *Neurology,* 1960;10:555-563.
[20] Ellrich J, Andersen OK, Messlinger K, Arendt-Nielsen L. Convergence of meningeal and facial afferents onto trigeminal brainstem neurons: an electrophysiological study in rat and man. *Pain,* 1999;82:229-237.
[21] Northfield D. Some observations on headache. *Brain*, 1938;61:133-162.
[22] Fay T. Atypical facial neuralgia, a syndrome of vascular pain. *Ann. Otol.,* 1932;41:1030-1062.
[23] Ferrari MD, Saxena PR. Clinical and experimental effects of sumatriptan in humans. *Trends Pharmacol. Sci.*, 1993;14:129-133.
[24] Shevel E. The extracranial vascular theory of migraine--a great story confirmed by the facts. *Headache,* 2011;51:409-417.
[25] Levy D, Burstein R. The vascular theory of migraine: leave it or love it? *Ann. Neurol.*, 2011;69:600-601.
[26] Ferro JM, Canhao P, Stam J, Bousser MG, Barinagarrementeria F. Prognosis of cerebral vein and dural sinus thrombosis: results of the International Study on Cerebral Vein and Dural Sinus Thrombosis (ISCVT). *Stroke,* 2004;35:664-670.
[27] Fontanarosa PB. Recognition of subarachnoid hemorrhage. *Ann. Emerg. Med.,* 1989;18:1199-1205.
[28] Massaro AR, Sacco RL, Mohr JP, et al. Clinical discriminators of lobar and deep hemorrhages: the Stroke Data Bank. *Neurology,* 1991;41:1881-1885.
[29] Rothrock JF. Headaches due to vascular disorders. *Neurol. Clin.* 2004;22:21-37, v.
[30] Silbert PL, Mokri B, Schievink WI. Headache and neck pain in spontaneous internal carotid and vertebral artery dissections. *Neurology,* 1995;45:1517-1522.
[31] Ducros A, Boukobza M, Porcher R, Sarov M, Valade D, Bousser MG. The clinical and radiological spectrum of reversible cerebral vasoconstriction syndrome. A prospective series of 67 patients. *Brain,* 2007;130:3091-3101.
[32] Sattar A, Manousakis G, Jensen MB. Systematic review of reversible cerebral vasoconstriction syndrome. *Expert Rev. Cardiovasc. Ther.*, 2011;8:1417-1421.
[33] Edmeads J. The headache of ischemic cerebrovascular disease. *Headache,* 1979;19:345-349.
[34] Ferro JM, Melo TP, Oliveira V, et al. A multivariate study of headache associated with ischemic stroke. *Headache,* 1995;35:315-319.
[35] Willinsky RA, Taylor SM, TerBrugge K, Farb RI, Tomlinson G, Montanera W. Neurologic complications of cerebral angiography: prospective analysis of 2,899 procedures and review of the literature. *Radiology,* 2003;227:522-528.
[36] Dawkins AA, Evans AL, Wattam J, et al. Complications of cerebral angiography: a prospective analysis of 2,924 consecutive procedures. *Neuroradiology,* 2007;49:753-759.

[37] Cloft HJ, Joseph GJ, Dion JE. Risk of cerebral angiography in patients with subarachnoid hemorrhage, cerebral aneurysm, and arteriovenous malformation: a meta-analysis. *Stroke,* 1999;30:317-320.
[38] Patterson RH, Jr., Goodell H, Dunning HS. Complications of Carotid Arteriography. *Arch. Neurol.*, 1964;10:513-520.
[39] Kaufmann TJ, Huston J, 3rd, Mandrekar JN, Schleck CD, Thielen KR, Kallmes DF. Complications of diagnostic cerebral angiography: evaluation of 19,826 consecutive patients. *Radiology,* 2007;243:812-819.
[40] Gil-Gouveia R, Fernandes Sousa R, Lopes L, Campos J, Pavao Martins I. Headaches during angiography and endovascular procedures. *J. Neurol.*, 2007;254:591-596.
[41] Hauge T. Catheter vertebral angiography. *Acta. Radiol. Suppl.,* 1954;109:1-219.
[42] Hauge T. Vertebral artery angiography and migraine-like symptoms: Hauge's studies reconsidered. *Cephalalgia,* 1986;6:197-203.
[43] Shuaib A, Hachinski VC. Migraine and the risks from angiography. *Arch. Neurol.*, 1988;45:911-912.
[44] Nichols FT, 3rd, Mawad M, Mohr JP, Stein B, Hilal S, Michelsen WJ. Focal headache during balloon inflation in the internal carotid and middle cerebral arteries. *Stroke,* 1990;21:555-559.
[45] Martins IP, Baeta E, Paiva T, Campos J, Gomes L. Headaches during intracranial endovascular procedures: a possible model of vascular headache. *Headache,* 1993;33:227-233.
[46] Nichols FT, 3rd, Mawad M, Mohr JP, Hilal S, Adams RJ. Focal headache during balloon inflation in the vertebral and basilar arteries. *Headache,* 1993;33:87-89.
[47] Munari LM, Belloni G, Moschini L, Mauro A, Pezzuoli G, Porta M. Carotid pain during percutaneous angioplasty (PTA). Pathophysiology and clinical features. *Cephalalgia,* 1994;14:127-131.
[48] Broman T, Olsson O. Experimental study of contrast media for cerebral angiography with reference to possible injurious effects on the cerebral blood vessels. *Acta. Radiol.*, 1949;31:321-334.
[49] Gil-Gouveia R, Martins IP. Headache and Angiography Study (data not published). In, 2007-2008.
[50] Gil-Gouveia RS, Sousa RF, Lopes L, Campos J, Martins IP. Post-angiography headaches. *J. Headache Pain.,* 2008;9:327-330.
[51] Takigawa T, Matsumaru Y, Nakai Y, et al. Bioactive Coils Cause Headache and Fever After Endovascular Treatment of Intracranial Aneurysms. *Headache,* 2011.
[52] Ramadan NM, Gilkey SJ, Mitchell M, Sawaya KL, Mitsias P. Postangiography headache. *Headache,* 1995;35:21-24.
[53] Beekman R, Nijssen PC, van Rooij WJ, Wijnalda D. Migraine with aura after intracranial endovascular procedures. *Headache,* 2001;41:410-413.
[54] Olsen TS, Johansen AM, Skriver E, Herning MG. [Migraine with aura (classical migraine) in patients examined for cerebrovascular disease]. *Ugeskr. Laeger.*, 1990;152:1513-1515.
[55] Kremer S, Grand S, Dananchet Y, et al. MRI during postangiography headache. *Neurology,* 2002;58:1425.
[56] Choxi AA, Durrani AK, Mericle RA. Both surgical clipping and endovascular embolization of unruptured intracranial aneurysms are associated with long-term

improvement in self-reported quantitative headache scores. *Neurosurgery,* 2011;69:128-133; discussion 133-124.

[57] The International Classification of Headache Disorders: 2nd edition. *Cephalalgia,* 2004;24 Suppl 1:9-160.

In: New Developments in Angiography Research
Editors: K. I. Sanders and A. M. Jackson
ISBN: 978-1-62081-492-5

Chapter VI

A New Horizon for Coronary Surgery: Hybrid Coronary Revascularization and Routine Intra-Operative Completion Angiography

Marzia Leacche[1], Annemarie Thompson[2], David X. Zhao[3], Bernhard J. Riedel[2] and John G. Byrne[1]

[1]Department of Cardiac Surgery, Vanderbilt Heart and Vascular Institute, Vanderbilt University, Nashville, TN, US

[2]Department of Anesthesiology, Vanderbilt Heart and Vascular Institute, Vanderbilt University, Nashville, TN, US

[3]Department of Cardiology, Vanderbilt Heart and Vascular Institute, Vanderbilt University, Nashville, TN, US

Abstract

Hybrid coronary revascularization combines coronary artery bypass grafting (CABG) surgery with percutaneous coronary intervention (PCI) for coronary artery disease. Surgical grafting is reserved for revascularization of the left anterior descending (LAD) artery, usually performed with the left internal mammary artery (LIMA) through either a limited thoracotomy or an endoscopic approach, while PCI with stenting is reserved for revascularization of non-LAD lesions. This combines the benefits of each technique—namely, the superiority of the LIMA to LAD graft and the improved patency rate of stent placement in non-LAD vessels. For non-LAD vessels, the higher one-year failure rate for saphenous vein grafts (SVG, averages 20%) compared to drug-eluting stents (DES, average 9%) supports this hybrid approach.

The hybrid procedure can be performed as a staged procedure—with PCI followed by CABG or CABG followed by PCI. However, hybrid coronary revascularization is increasingly performed as a combined ("one stop") procedure in a dedicated suite—the "hybrid operating room". The hybrid room has the capability of serving both as a complete surgical operating room and as a catheterization laboratory.

The hybrid operating room also allows for routine completion angiography following CABG surgery. This facilitates early identification of graft failure thereby providing the opportunity to correct technical errors within the same surgical period and thus may improve graft patency rate, especially of SVG to non-LAD vessels. This chapter reviews the advantages of and the logistics required for performing hybrid procedures and completion angiography—a new horizon for coronary surgery.

Keywords: Coronary artery bypass grafting surgery; hybrid coronary revascularization; coronary angiography; percutaneous coronary intervention

INTRODUCTION

Current therapeutic strategies for managing coronary artery disease include medical therapy, percutaneous coronary intervention (PCI) and coronary artery bypass grafting (CABG) surgery.

Several trials compared outcomes after CABG surgery versus PCI for multi-vessel coronary artery disease, with the BARI, ARTS and SoS trials all reporting a survival benefit following CABG surgery in diabetic patients. [1-4] However, in the non-diabetic population, the impact on survival remains questionable with the ARTS trial [4] reporting a 5-year survival similar for revascularization with CABG and PCI while the SoS trial [1] reported an improved 5-year survival following CABG surgery. Importantly, the ARTS trial found an increased need for repeat revascularization in the PCI group (30.3% vs. 8.8%).

Drug eluting stents (DES) have a lower re-stenosis rate than bare metal stents (BMS). In fact, the 12-18 month re-stenosis rate for DES (8.6% in the SIRIUS study with sirolimus stents and 11% in the TAXUS 1 and ASPECT trials with paclitaxel stents) [5-10] is lower than the occlusion rate for saphenous vein grafts (SVG; average 20%, range 1.6% to 30%). [11-13] DES therefore have the potential to provide better long-term results than that seen with vein grafts.

Hybrid coronary revascularization combines PCI (DES for non-LAD lesions) with CABG surgery (LIMA to LAD graft). The LIMA to LAD graft can be performed utilizing one of three approaches: a standard sternotomy approach, a Minimally Invasive Direct Coronary Artery Bypass (MIDCAB; antero-lateral mini-thoracotomy) approach, or a Totally Endoscopic Coronary Artery Bypass (TECAB) approach. With TECAB, the LIMA to LAD graft is crafted with a robotic system using thoracic ports and then PCI to the remaining left and right coronary arteries (Figure 1A and 1B).

Hybrid procedures can be staged with an interval spanning days or weeks. Alternatively, this is increasingly performed in a single session utilizing a dedicated suite, the hybrid operating room (OR)—a fully equipped catheterization suite integrated with a fully equipped operating room. This procedural suite allows "one stop" hybrid revascularization. Additionally, this hybrid suite provides for intra-operative assessment of surgical bypass graft integrity.

The importance of this lies in the fact that early graft failure, largely related to technical errors at the time of the surgery, can now be assessed and potentially corrected in a timely fashion. While it is standard of care to perform completion imaging at the end of valve surgery, PCI and repair of congenital defects, post-procedural imaging is not routine for CABG surgery. We envision the hybrid OR will expand the indication for completion imaging to include CABG surgery.

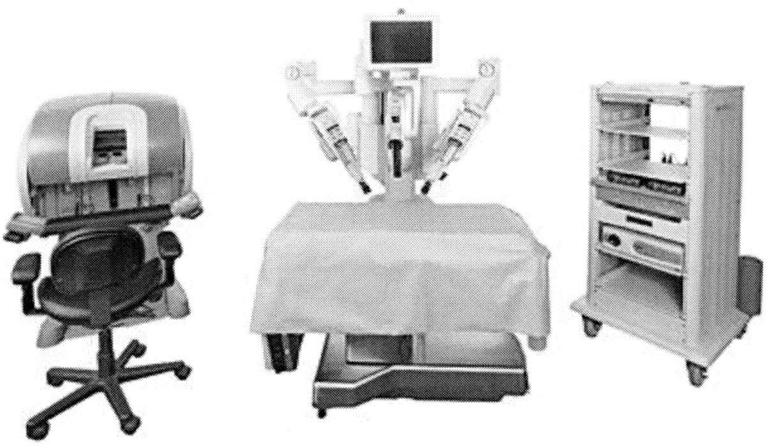

Figure 1A. The Da Vinci Surgical S system, with the surgeon's console, the robot and the components (*©2008 Intuitive Surgical, Inc).*

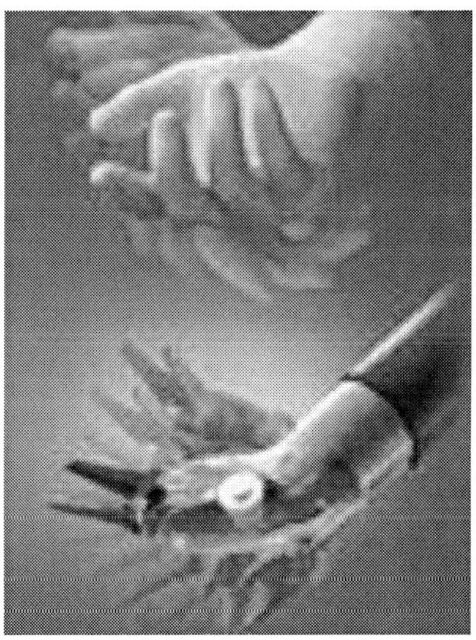

Figure 1B. EndoWrist® and Surgeon Hands (© 2008 Intuitive Surgical, Inc).

INTRA-OPERATIVE IMAGING FOR CABG SURGERY

Revascularization with CABG surgery is a lifesaving procedure with long-term benefits dependant upon graft patency. A recent multicenter randomized study (3,041 patients) reported a 13.9% incidence of combined endpoints (death and new myocardial infarction) in patients with one or more occluded SVGs (vs. 0.9% incidence in those patients with patent SVGs). [12] Since early graft failure is mainly caused by technical errors at the time of surgery, a number of methods are currently used to assess graft integrity in the OR. Intra-operative graft patency is inferred using indirect signs such as the presence of graft pulsation, the absence of hemodynamic instability, electrocardiographic changes or new regional wall motion abnormality on echocardiography. These methods have varying reliability, and hemodynamic compromise or electrocardiographic changes may be absent even in the presence of complete graft occlusion. [13] This 'silent' ischemia is attributed to factors such as the location of the coronary vessel, the grade of native coronary artery disease, the myocardial territory supplied, and the existence of collateral blood flow. In our experience of 796 grafts imaged in the hybrid operating room with 97 (12%) grafts having a demonstrable angiographic defect, only a few patients demonstrated hemodynamic instability and/or electrocardiographic changes, while most, despite having a significant graft defect, did not.(reference JACC paper here). Currently the most common method to assess intra-operative graft patency is transit time flow measurement (TTFM), a quantitative volume flow Doppler technique which measures blood flow through the bypassed myocardial vessel.

The advantage is that TTFM can be measured in any OR not equipped with imaging capability. D'Ancona et al., [14] in a large series of patients, reported a 3.2% revision rate after TTFM was used to assess graft patency—a rate well below the 1-year SVG failure rate (20%). [13] Compared to TTFM, coronary angiography can identify higher rate of occluded grafts. [15, 16]

Limitations of TTFM include: inability to define the degree of stenosis, inability to discriminate the influence of the graft conduit from that of the coronary arteriolar bed, and variability in normal flow data which is dependant upon several factors (including: systemic arterial pressure, cardiac output, peripheral vascular resistance, type of graft used [vein conduit vs. arterial conduit], residual antegrade coronary flow, resistance of the distal coronary bed, competitive native flow and hematocrit).

Intra-operative fluorescence imaging (IFI; Novadaq Technologies Inc., Toronto, Canada) has been more recently introduced to assess intra-operative graft patency. Using this technique, Taggart et al. [17] identified 1.9% of graft failure in 213 grafts imaged.

Compared to TTFM, the IFI has superior sensitivity and specificity to detect an occlusion of 50% or more in the imaged graft. [18[However, IFI provides a semi-quantitative rather than a detailed assessment of the anastomosis. Moreover, the transit of the green dye is dependant upon several factors (including: conduit diameter, native coronary bed resistance, competitive native coronary flow, systemic arterial pressure, and hematocrit) and thus normal values can also vary considerably.

For the abovementioned reasons, coronary angiography remains the gold standard to assess graft patency. To date, the major limiting factors to performing completion angiography after CABG surgery has been the need of a specially designed 'hybrid' OR and increased cooperation among cardiologists and cardiac surgeons.

The Hybrid Operating Room

The hybrid OR requires more space than a standard catheterization suite or operating room and is more expensive to build (Figure 2, shows a hybrid OR at Vanderbilt University Medical Center—one of the first in the US). However, this multifunctional OR can be utilized as a fully functional catheterization suite, as an endovascular procedural suite, as an electrophysiology suite, or as a fully equipped OR thereby ensuring optimal use of this resource. An added advantage of a hybrid OR is the real-time collaboration between the interventional and OR teams, with synergy in teamwork that promotes a high level of trust between cardiac surgeons and cardiologists.

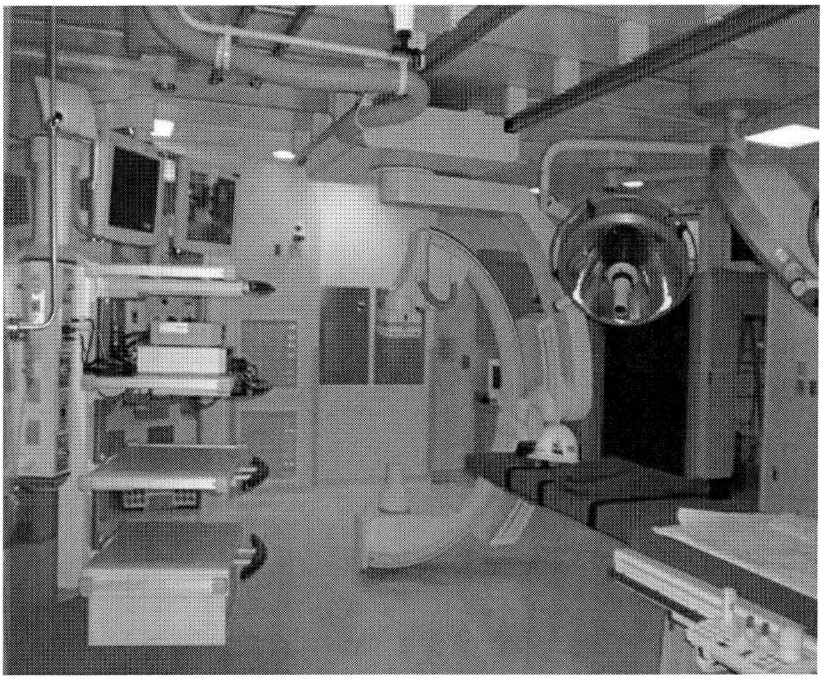

Figure 2. The Vanderbilt hybrid operating room.

The following provides a synopsis of our experience (796 grafts imaged before chest closure in 366 patients [71] with completion angiography in the hybrid OR at Vanderbilt University Medical Center. Before heparinization for CABG, a femoral sheath is placed in the femoral artery using the Seldinger technique. For off-pump (OPCAB, MIDCAB) and on-pump CABG surgery, heparin (150 IU·kg-1 or 300 IU·kg-1, respectively) is dosed to achieve an adequate activated clotting time (ACT; >250 seconds or >400 seconds, respectively). After completion of bypass grafting (and weaning from cardiopulmonary bypass with decannulation following on-pump surgery) the heparin is fully reversed with protamine. The open sternal wound is covered with a triple layer (two towels and one large surgical drape) prior to moving the camera into place over the open chest. The camera itself is covered by a double drape, once prior to movement and again upon arrival over the patient (Figure 3). A completion angiogram is then done by an interventional cardiologist. Once a satisfactory result is confirmed, the chest incision is closed, the femoral sheath is removed, hemostasis is obtained with a vascular closure device and manual compression, and the patient is transferred to the intensive care unit for postoperative management. Relative contraindications for intra-operative completion angiography include the presence of significant plaque burden (grade 4-5 atheroma—plaque protruding >5mm into the aortic lumen or any size with a mobile component as defined by transesophageal echocardiography) in the aortic arch or descending thoracic aorta and the presence of renal dysfunction (our arbitrary cut off value is creatinine ≥2 mg·dL-1).

Our data suggest a 4% incidence of new onset acute renal failure (defined as a 2-fold increase in serum creatinine relative to the preoperative value) and 1% incidence of requirement for postoperative dialysis. These rates correspond with the reported incidence of acute renal failure following CABG surgery. [19]

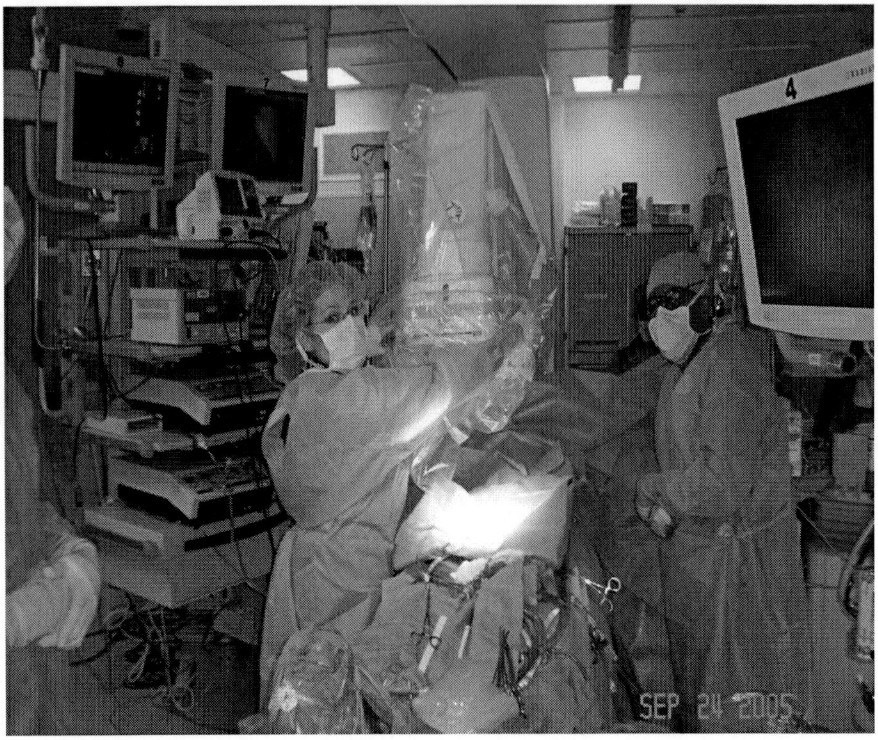

Figure 3. The draping of the C-arm in the hybrid operating room.

Hybrid Procedures

The 10-year patency rate for LIMA to LAD grafting is estimated at between 95% and 98%. [20, 21] Such high patency rates for LIMA grafts translate into excellent patient outcomes with reduced risk of death, myocardial infarction, recurrent angina, and need for further revascularization. [22, 23] Conversely, the re-stenosis rate for PCI performed to the LAD is estimated between 19% - 44%. [24, 25] Head-to-head comparisons of LIMA to LAD grafting versus PCI for proximal LAD lesions was performed predominantly with bare metal stents. [26, 27]

A meta-analysis [28] of six randomized trials comparing PCI and MIDCAB (LIMA to LAD) reported that the combined end-point of mortality, myocardial infarction and target vessel revascularization was significantly higher (RR=2.27; 95%CI 1.32, 3.90; p=0.003) in the PCI group. However, only one of the six studies used DES and the results may not be representative of current medical practice. Recent data provide conflicting results: some studies report no difference in major adverse cardiac events or requirement for repeat revascularization at 6-12 month follow-up, [29, 30] while other studies report superior outcomes for CABG surgery. [31, 32]

The discrepancy among these studies reflects differences in terms of the type of lesion treated, presence of multivessel disease and use of DES versus BMS. Sub-analyses from the TAXUS IV [33] and SIRIUS [34] studies suggest that lower rates of target lesion revascularization (TLR; 5.8% versus 16.7 %; p <0.001 for TAXUS IV and 6.0% versus 23%; p <0.001 for SIRIUS) are required for DES versus bare metal stents, with 13.5% and 9.8%

incidence of major adverse cardiac events at 1-year follow-up was for the TAXUS IV and SIRIUS studies, respectively.

The second conduit of choice for CABG surgery is the SVG. Despite advances in surgical technique a high rate of SVG failure is still reported in the present era of CABG surgery. In fact, the PREVENT IV trial reported a concerning 30% SVG failure rate at 1 year follow-up. [12]

This unexpected high failure rate has not been fully explained, with technical errors during surgery being one possible reason contributing to SVG failure. However, other factors may also include poor quality conduit and poor distal targets.

Assessing vein graft quality in the OR typically relies on visual inspection. In our experience of 439 vein grafts imaged [71] we observed a high rate of SVG to coronary artery mismatch (where-in the size of the vein conduit was much larger than that of the coronary vessel; Figure 4), minor (to the naked eye) kinks, and the presence of vein valve's which can limit the antegrade flow.

The long-term impact of these angiographic findings is currently under investigation, but to date remains largely unknown. For all the above reasons, revascularization with SVGs may have a lower patency rate than with DES. Thus, depending upon the quality of the coronary vessel and conduit, in selected patients a 'hybrid approach,' combining LIMA to LAD graft with DES for the right coronary artery (RCA) and/or left circumflex (LCX) coronary artery systems, may be a better approach.

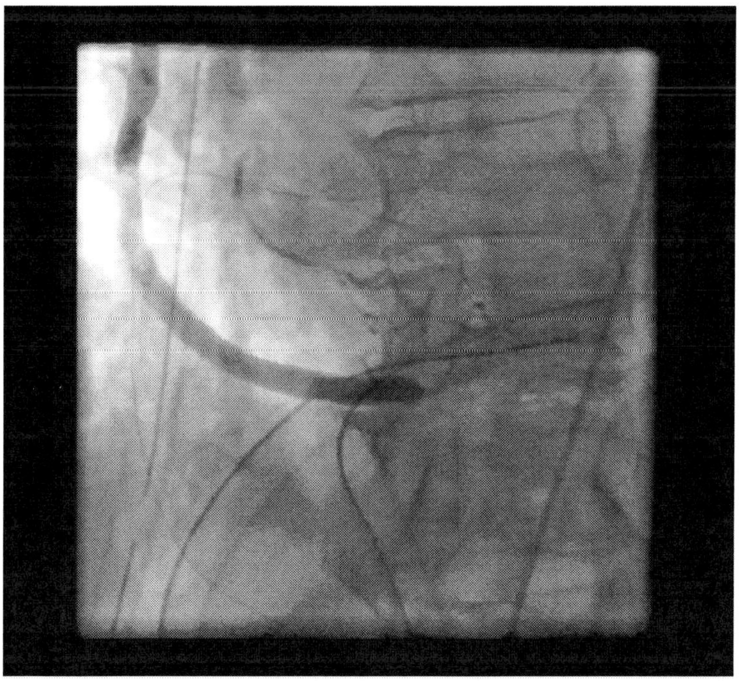

Figure 4. A saphenous vein graft to the posterior descending artery wherein the size of the vein conduit is much larger than that of the coronary vessel.

Indications and Contraindications for Hybrid CABG Surgery

Patients with a high-grade proximal lesion of the LAD and lesions favorable for PCI in the LCX and RCA territory are ideal candidates for hybrid coronary revascularization. Other potential indications for PCI as an alternative to SVG conduit include poor quality conduit (Figure 5), small or diffuse distal coronary artery disease with non graftable native coronary vessel that is still favorable for PCI (Figure 6), redo operations, severe atherosclerotic ascending aortic disease, and acute coronary syndromes.

Contraindications to performing MIDCAB and TECAB approaches include concomitant valvular disease, intramyocardial LAD artery, severe lung disease precluding single lung ventilation, subclavian artery stenosis, heart failure, and prior chest irradiation (relative). More specifically to TECAB, the presence of severe abdominal adhesions may preclude sub-xiphoid placement of the endostabilizer.

If the TECAB technique is performed with CPB then the presence of severe peripheral vascular disease is a contraindication because of the inability to institute femoral CPB. For the MIDCAB approach, morbid obesity may represent a relative contraindication. These techniques are usually performed in patients with stable coronary artery disease, as acute ischemic events may preclude procedures of longer duration.

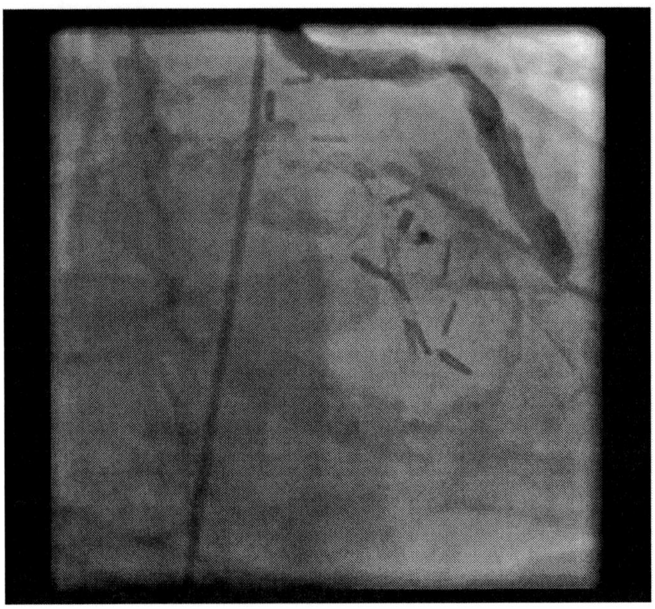

Figure 5. Poor conduit quality of a vein graft at completion angiogram.

Results and Limitations of Hybrid Coronary Revascularization

The first hybrid coronary revascularization was performed in 1996, with six patients having revascularization with a LIMA to LAD though an antero-lateral mini-thoracotomy and then PCI/PTCA to non LAD lesions. [35] Since 1996, hybrid coronary revascularization has been adopted by several groups and is performed with low mortality (0% - 2%), low transfusion rate, absence of neurologic complications, superior cosmetic results, and faster recovery than conventional CABG surgery. [36-54] These series report a variable range in in-hospital morbidity (0% - 21%, average of 5%). [36, 41] Despite these favorable results, hybrid CABG surgery has not become popular and the largest series of hybrid CABG cases to date only accounts for 70 patients. [46] Contributory factors may include the perceived technical difficulty associated with MIDCAB/TECAB procedures—mostly related to difficulty in stabilizing the target vessel—resulting in concern for the anastomotic quality and thus patency rate. In experienced centers, the immediate LIMA patency rates (within 6 months) vary between 92% - 100%. [38, 45] These results, however, may not necessarily be reproducible. Goldstein et al. [55] reported a 42% incidence of anastomotic defects and 35% incidence of LIMA arterial spasm in their experience of 26 MIDCAB procedures. Further, the concern for requirement of repeat revascularization related to stent restenosis after PCI is a further limiting factor. Importantly, the studies reporting on PCI in hybrid series frequently utilized BMS and PTCA in the past. [36-40, 54] Thus, as stent technology improves the "re-interventional gap" between surgery (SVG) and DES may decrease. [33,34] In fact, a recent series reporting on 15 hybrid (CABG/PCI) patients reported a 97% 1-year patency rate for the DES. [47]

Timing of Hybrid Coronary Revascularization

Hybrid coronary revascularization can be performed either in a staged fashion or in a "one stop" setting in which the patient undergoes PCI and surgery in the hybrid OR. In the staged hybrid procedure, PCI can be performed either before or after CABG surgery. If PCI is performed before CABG surgery, it permits aggressive multivessel stenting and in the event of a complication or failure, CABG will be performed at a later stage. Due to the antiplatelet regimen required for patients who undergo PCI and stenting, drawbacks to stenting prior to coronary surgery include the need to operate on patients requiring clopidogrel therapy and the lack of angiographic assessment of the bypass graft postoperatively. However, if PCI is done after CABG surgery then the LIMA to LAD graft can be assessed at the time of PCI. Additionally, this sequence also reduces the bleeding risk associated with clopidogrel therapy instituted with stent placement. If angiography during PCI reveals a PCI-related complication or LIMA to LAD graft patency issues then medical therapy, revision of grafts or reoperation can be performed prior to leaving the operating room. Centers that practice staged hybrid procedures prefer the latter sequence—to perform CABG first followed by PCI.

At the Vanderbilt University Medical Center we have performed 112 "one stop" hybrid procedures. [71] In our opinion, this approach may be a superior to a staged procedure since complications associated with PCI or CABG surgery can be identified immediately and prompt surgical or percutaneous revision of compromised grafts done. Additionally, early graft patency can be verified at completion of the initial surgery. In the presence of a graft problem, PCI provides a valuable alternative to surgery for revising the graft defect. Moreover, this strategy avoids the logistic burden and time delay inherent to a staged procedure.

For hybrid procedures where percutaneous coronary intervention is planned, patients receive preoperative clopidogrel to minimize the incidence of in-stent thrombosis. Adverse reactions to protamine and the theoretical potential for stent thrombosis should be carefully considered during reversal of anticoagulation with protamine. Although we currently reverse with a full dose of protamine, a reduced dose may be required for complex stent procedures that necessitate judicious antiplatelet therapy. The possible increased blood loss in patients who undergo cardiac surgery while taking clopidogrel should be anticipated and monitored. Conflicting data exist with regards to the incidence of increased bleeding in hybrid procedures. [47, 53, 56] In our experience, we found increased chest tube output drainage but the rate of reoperation for bleeding was similar between hybrid and standard CABG patients.

Timing of clopidogrel administration in an attempt to balance the risk of bleeding with the prevention of DES thrombosis is important. Maximal inhibition of platelet aggregation occurs after 4 - 24 hours. [57, 58] In our current practice, if a hybrid procedure is planned we load patients with 300 mg of clopidogrel (rather than 600 mg to decrease the risk of bleeding) in the immediate preoperative period prior to surgery. In those patients where stents are placed in response to an intraoperative graft defect identified at completion angiography (unplanned hybrid), the clopidogrel is administered through a orogastric tube either prior to stent placement or immediately after the completion of surgery. The rate of absorption of clopidogrel through the orogastric tube under general anesthesia, the unknown effects of heparin reversal with protamine on stent patency, and the interaction of clopidogrel on cardiopulmonary bypass-induced platelet and coagulation cascade dysfunction require further investigation.

Contrast Nephropathy

A particular concern for patient undergoing hybrid coronary revascularization is the incidence of hospital-acquired nephropathy, with risk of contrast-induced nephropathy (CIN) following coronary angiography. CIN is a concern following routine completion angiography and following hybrid procedures, since contrast agent exposure and cardiac surgery are known major risk factors for hospital acquired nephropathy. Although the risk of CIN in around 2% in healthy adults, the risk is increased in patients with diabetes mellitus, pre-existing renal dysfunction, heart failure, dehydration, previous diuretic use, hypoalbuminemia, increased age, and increased contrast volume. [59, 60,61] In these high risk patients, the incidence of CIN may be as high as 15%. [59, 62] Several studies have sought to identify possible preventive therapies for CIN, such as sodium bicarbonate, normal saline hydration, and N-acetylcysteine.

To date, the most effective strategies for prevention of CIN are minimizing contrast volume, use of iso-osmolar contrast, and preprocedural hydration. [63] The preferred fluid for prehydration is normal saline rather than half-normal saline, as suggested by a large randomized controlled trial. [64] The addition of N-acetycysteine to the preprocedural hydration is often added to prevent CIN, although there is conflicting data regarding the added benefit of N-acetylcysteine to hydration alone. [64-66]

We and other groups have documented the safety of completion angiography following CABG surgery without an increased risk for acquired postoperative nephropathy. Risks factors currently associated with postoperative nephropathy after CABG surgery include age and elevated preoperative serum creatinine. [67]

No correlation has been found between the dose of contrast agent (iodixanol) and the incidence of CIN. [67] Completion angiography requires a median amount of 150 mL (range:

20-500mL) of contrast agent, which is comparable to that used for computed tomography. Hybrid patients (those who undergo PCI) usually require a larger dose. In our experience, the incidence of acute renal failure (defined as a doubling of the serum creatinine from baseline value) was similar (2.6% vs. 3.9%; p = NS) when hybrid and non hybrid patients were compared.

Anesthetic Considerations for Hybrid Coronary Procedures

Hybrid coronary revascularization procedures require the skill and experience of cardiac anesthesiologists during the planning and execution phases of a hybrid OR. Surgical capability combined with cardiovascular imaging with transesophageal echocardiography (TEE) and coronary angiography create a unique environment for a breadth of cardiovascular procedures, including, but not limited to, hybrid coronary revascularization. Endovascular repair of prosthetic perivalvular leaks with Amplatzer devices, high-risk (left main stem) percutaneous interventions in patients deemed to be poor surgical candidates, and laser removal of pacemaker/defibrillator leads are other examples of procedures performed in the highly specialized but versatile environment of a hybrid operating room. The cardiac anesthesiologist must understand the specific anesthetic and medical implications of these procedures while working in an environment with multiple proceduralists caring for the same patient.

If the hybrid OR is in the cardiac catheterization area and not in the surgical operating area, the cardiac anesthesiologist must recognize that the delivery of safe patient care requires that it be considered a "remote location", meaning the physical location of the hybrid OR is away from other surgical areas. Recommendations for monitoring and technical support for remote locations are detailed elsewhere. [68] Although cardiovascular patients undergoing cardiac surgery are not represented in published descriptions of patient populations in remote locations, our clinical series and the experience of other centers report no increase in morbidity and mortality for hybrid coronary procedures. However, the prerequisites for successful, safe coronary revascularization procedures may be more detailed than those required for anesthetic management of more traditional remote location procedures, due to the highly invasive nature of CABG surgery and the co-morbidities associated with cardiac surgery patients, who are typically class 3-5 according to the American Society of Anesthesiologists Physical Status Classification System.

Essential anesthetic equipment includes, but is not limited to, an anesthetic machine with necessary gas lines, a scavenging system, and an anesthetic cart with medicines and supplies commonly used in cardiac anesthesia. [69] In addition, specialized airway equipment should be immediately available in the event of an unanticipated difficult airway. Even with the availability of cardiac catheterization in the hybrid OR, TEE is an indispensable skill in cardiac anesthesia, and a TEE machine is essential. Invasive monitoring is also required for these procedures; therefore, central venous access catheters as well as arterial catheters should be available. Due to the possible increased transit time for laboratory blood samples from remote locations as well as the frequency and urgency of laboratory testing in the critically ill cardiac surgery patients, a system of obtaining rapid laboratory results, such as point-of-care testing should be considered. Since the transfusion rate of cardiac surgery patients is typically 40 - 70% in some series and hemodynamic medications are often required, a system of rapid order entry and efficient transport of blood products and medications should be anticipated and established before hybrid coronary revascularization procedures are performed. [70]

Conclusion

CABG surgery is currently the only procedure performed in cardiac surgery without intraoperative imaging. Methods (TTFM and IFI) used to assess graft patency and the quality of the coronary anastomosis offer limited detection of graft defects. Intraoperative completion angiography may improve detection of these defects allowing timely intervention and thereby reduce the incidence of early graft failure.

Hybrid coronary revascularization is feasible and safe and is currently performed in a few centers predominantly for high-risk patients unsuitable for PCI or CABG surgery alone. With the advent of newer and better performing stents, with lower rates of re-stenosis, PCI may offer superior revascularization of non-LAD vessels than that currently achieved with SVG. It is anticipated that hybrid coronary revascularization will be increasingly adopted, especially since the complexity of patients has increased. With more elderly patients presenting with diffuse coronary artery disease, often with previous multi-vessel stenting, the ability to revascularize with less invasive approaches is appealing.

References

[1] Coronary artery bypass surgery versus percutaneous coronary intervention with stent implantation in patients with multivessel coronary artery disease (the Stent or Surgery trial): a randomised controlled trial. *Lancet.* 2002;360(9338):965-970.

[2] The final 10-year follow-up results from the BARI randomized trial. *J. Am. Coll. Cardiol.* 2007;49(15):1600-1606.

[3] Hoffman SN, TenBrook JA, Wolf MP, Pauker SG, Salem DN, Wong JB. A meta-analysis of randomized controlled trials comparing coronary artery bypass graft with percutaneous transluminal coronary angioplasty: one- to eight-year outcomes. *J. Am. Coll. Cardiol.* 2003;41(8):1293-1304.

[4] Serruys PW, Ong AT, van Herwerden LA, Sousa JE, Jatene A, Bonnier JJ, Schonberger JP, Buller N, Bonser R, Disco C, Backx B, Hugenholtz PG, Firth BG, Unger F. Five-year outcomes after coronary stenting versus bypass surgery for the treatment of multivessel disease: the final analysis of the Arterial Revascularization Therapies Study (ARTS) randomized trial. *J. Am. Coll. Cardiol.* 2005;46(4):575-581.

[5] Flynn TC, Ma J. Theoretical analysis of twist/bend ratio and mechanical moduli of bacterial flagellar hook and filament. *Biophys. J.* 2004;86(5):3204-3210.

[6] Park SJ, Shim WH, Ho DS, Raizner AE, Park SW, Hong MK, Lee CW, Choi D, Jang Y, Lam R, Weissman NJ, Mintz GS. A paclitaxel-eluting stent for the prevention of coronary restenosis. *N. Engl. J. Med.* 2003;348(16):1537-1545.

[7] Moses JW, Leon MB, Popma JJ, Fitzgerald PJ, Holmes DR, O'Shaughnessy C, Caputo RP, Kereiakes DJ, Williams DO, Teirstein PS, Jaeger JL, Kuntz RE. Sirolimus-eluting

stents versus standard stents in patients with stenosis in a native coronary artery. *N. Engl. J. Med.* 2003;349(14):1315-1323.

[8] Grube E, Silber S, Hauptmann KE, Mueller R, Buellesfeld L, Gerckens U, Russell ME. TAXUS I: six- and twelve-month results from a randomized, double-blind trial on a slow-release paclitaxel-eluting stent for de novo coronary lesions. *Circulation.* 2003;107(1):38-42.

[9] Murphy GJ, Bryan AJ, Angelini GD. Hybrid coronary revascularization in the era of drug-eluting stents. *Ann. Thorac. Surg.* 2004;78(5):1861-1867.

[10] Schampaert E, Moses JW, Schofer J, Schluter M, Gershlick AH, Cohen EA, Palisaitis DA, Breithardt G, Donohoe DJ, Wang H, Popma JJ, Kuntz RE, Leon MB. Sirolimus-eluting stents at two years: a pooled analysis of SIRIUS, E-SIRIUS, and C-SIRIUS with emphasis on late revascularizations and stent thromboses. *Am. J. Cardiol.* 2006;98(1): 36-41.

[11] Nathoe HM, van Dijk D, Jansen EW, Suyker WJ, Diephuis JC, van Boven WJ, de la Riviere AB, Borst C, Kalkman CJ, Grobbee DE, Buskens E, de Jaegere PP. A comparison of on-pump and off-pump coronary bypass surgery in low-risk patients. *N. Engl. J. Med.* 2003;348(5):394-402.

[12] Alexander JH, Hafley G, Harrington RA, Peterson ED, Ferguson TB, Jr., Lorenz TJ, Goyal A, Gibson M, Mack MJ, Gennevois D, Califf RM, Kouchoukos NT. Efficacy and safety of edifoligide, an E2F transcription factor decoy, for prevention of vein graft failure following coronary artery bypass graft surgery: PREVENT IV: a randomized controlled trial. *Jama.* 2005;294(19):2446-2454.

[13] Balacumaraswami L, Taggart DP. Intraoperative imaging techniques to assess coronary artery bypass graft patency. *Ann. Thorac. Surg.* 2007;83(6):2251-2257.

[14] D'Ancona G, Karamanoukian HL, Ricci M, Schmid S, Bergsland J, Salerno TA. Graft revision after transit time flow measurement in off-pump coronary artery bypass grafting. *Eur. J. Cardiothorac. Surg.* 2000;17(3):287-293.

[15] Hol PK, Lingaas PS, Lundblad R, Rein KA, Vatne K, Smith HJ, Nitter-Hauge S, Fosse E. Intraoperative angiography leads to graft revision in coronary artery bypass surgery. *Ann. Thorac. Surg.* 2004;78(2):502-505; discussion 505.

[16] Hirotani T, Kameda T, Shirota S, Nakao Y. An evaluation of the intraoperative transit time measurements of coronary bypass flow. *Eur. J. Cardiothorac. Surg.* 2001;19(6):848-852.

[17] Taggart DP, Choudhary B, Anastasiadis K, Abu-Omar Y, Balacumaraswami L, Pigott DW. Preliminary experience with a novel intraoperative fluorescence imaging technique to evaluate the patency of bypass grafts in total arterial revascularization. *Ann. Thorac. Surg.* 2003;75(3):870-873.

[18] Desai ND, Miwa S, Kodama D, Koyama T, Cohen G, Pelletier MP, Cohen EA, Christakis GT, Goldman BS, Fremes SE. A randomized comparison of intraoperative indocyanine green angiography and transit-time flow measurement to detect technical errors in coronary bypass grafts. *J. Thorac. Cardiovasc. Surg.* 2006;132(3):585-594.

[19] Rosner MH, Okusa MD. Acute kidney injury associated with cardiac surgery. *Clin. J. Am. Soc. Nephrol.* 2006;1(1):19-32.

[20] Hayward PA, Buxton BF. Contemporary coronary graft patency: 5-year observational data from a randomized trial of conduits. *Ann. Thorac. Surg.* 2007;84(3):795-799.

[21] Tatoulis J, Buxton BF, Fuller JA. Patencies of 2127 arterial to coronary conduits over 15 years. *Ann. Thorac. Surg.* 2004;77(1):93-101.

[22] Yusuf S, Zucker D, Peduzzi P, Fisher LD, Takaro T, Kennedy JW, Davis K, Killip T, Passamani E, Norris R, et al. Effect of coronary artery bypass graft surgery on survival: overview of 10-year results from randomised trials by the Coronary Artery Bypass Graft Surgery Trialists Collaboration. *Lancet.* 1994;344(8922):563-570.

[23] Loop FD, Lytle BW, Cosgrove DM, Stewart RW, Goormastic M, Williams GW, Golding LA, Gill CC, Taylor PC, Sheldon WC, et al. Influence of the internal-mammary-artery graft on 10-year survival and other cardiac events. *N. Engl. J. Med.* 1986;314(1):1-6.

[24] Versaci F, Gaspardone A, Tomai F, Crea F, Chiariello L, Gioffre PA. A comparison of coronary-artery stenting with angioplasty for isolated stenosis of the proximal left anterior descending coronary artery. *N. Engl. J. Med.* 1997;336(12):817-822.

[25] Kastrati A, Schomig A, Elezi S, Schuhlen H, Dirschinger J, Hadamitzky M, Wehinger A, Hausleiter J, Walter H, Neumann FJ. Predictive factors of restenosis after coronary stent placement. *J. Am. Coll. Cardiol.* 1997;30(6):1428-1436.

[26] Goy JJ, Kaufmann U, Goy-Eggenberger D, Garachemani A, Hurni M, Carrel T, Gaspardone A, Burnand B, Meier B, Versaci F, Tomai F, Bertel O, Pieper M, de Benedictis M, Eeckhout E. A prospective randomized trial comparing stenting to internal mammary artery grafting for proximal, isolated de novo left anterior coronary artery stenosis: the SIMA trial. Stenting vs Internal Mammary Artery. *Mayo. Clin. Proc.* 2000;75(11):1116-1123.

[27] Drenth DJ, Veeger NJ, Winter JB, Grandjean JG, Mariani MA, Boven van AJ, Boonstra PW. A prospective randomized trial comparing stenting with off-pump coronary surgery for high-grade stenosis in the proximal left anterior descending coronary artery: three-year follow-up. *J. Am. Coll. Cardiol.* 2002;40(11):1955-1960.

[28] Jaffery Z, Kowalski M, Weaver WD, Khanal S. A meta-analysis of randomized control trials comparing minimally invasive direct coronary bypass grafting versus percutaneous coronary intervention for stenosis of the proximal left anterior descending artery. *Eur. J. Cardiothorac. Surg.* 2007;31(4):691-697.

[29] Hong SJ, Lim DS, Seo HS, Kim YH, Shim WJ, Park CG, Oh DJ, Ro YM. Percutaneous coronary intervention with drug-eluting stent implantation vs. minimally invasive direct coronary artery bypass (MIDCAB) in patients with left anterior descending coronary artery stenosis. *Catheter. Cardiovasc. Interv.* 2005;64(1):75-81.

[30] Reeves BC, Angelini GD, Bryan AJ, Taylor FC, Cripps T, Spyt TJ, Samani NJ, Roberts JA, Jacklin P, Seehra HK, Culliford LA, Keenan DJ, Rowlands DJ, Clarke B, Stanbridge R, Foale R. A multi-centre randomised controlled trial of minimally invasive direct coronary bypass grafting versus percutaneous transluminal coronary angioplasty with stenting for proximal stenosis of the left anterior descending coronary artery. *Health Technol. Assess.* 2004;8(16):1-43.

[31] Moshkovitz Y, Mohr R, Braunstein R, Zivi E, Uretzky G, Ben-Gal Y, Herz I. Revascularization of left anterior descending coronary artery in patients with single and multivessel disease: comparison between off-pump internal thoracic artery and drug-eluting stent. *Chest.* 2005;128(2):804-809.

[32] Herz I, Mohr R, Moshkovitz Y, Ben-Gal Y, Adam SZ, Braunstein R, Uretzky G. Revascularization of the left anterior descending artery with drug-eluting stents: comparison with arterial off-pump surgery. *Heart Surg. Forum.* 2004;7(5):E490-492.

[33] Dangas G, Ellis SG, Shlofmitz R, Katz S, Fish D, Martin S, Mehran R, Russell ME, Stone GW. Outcomes of paclitaxel-eluting stent implantation in patients with stenosis of the left anterior descending coronary artery. *J. Am. Coll. Cardiol.* 2005;45(8):1186-1192.

[34] Sawhney N, Moses JW, Leon MB, Kuntz RE, Popma JJ, Bachinsky W, Bass T, DeMaio S, Fry E, Holmes DR, Jr., Teirstein PS. Treatment of left anterior descending coronary artery disease with sirolimus-eluting stents. *Circulation.* 2004;110(4):374-379.

[35] Angelini GD, Wilde P, Salerno TA, Bosco G, Calafiore AM. Integrated left small thoracotomy and angioplasty for multivessel coronary artery revascularisation. *Lancet.* 1996;347(9003):757-758.

[36] Isomura T, Suma H, Horii T, Sato T, Kobashi T, Kanemitsu H. Minimally invasive coronary artery revascularization: off-pump bypass grafting and the hybrid procedure. *Ann. Thorac. Surg.* 2000;70(6):2017-2022.

[37] de Canniere D, Jansens JL, Goldschmidt-Clermont P, Barvais L, Decroly P, Stoupel E. Combination of minimally invasive coronary bypass and percutaneous transluminal coronary angioplasty in the treatment of double-vessel coronary disease: Two-year follow-up of a new hybrid procedure compared with "on-pump" double bypass grafting. *Am. Heart. J.* 2001;142(4):563-570.

[38] Presbitero P, Nicolini F, Maiello L, Franciosi G, Carcagni A, Milone F, Manasse E, Gallotti R. "Hybrid" percutaneous and surgical coronary revascularization: selection criteria from a single-center experience. *Ital. Heart. J.* 2001;2(5):363-368.

[39] Cisowski M, Morawski W, Drzewiecki J, Kruczak W, Toczek K, Bis J, Bochenek A. Integrated minimally invasive direct coronary artery bypass grafting and angioplasty for coronary artery revascularization. *Eur. J. Cardiothorac. Surg.* 2002;22(2):261-265.

[40] Stahl KD, Boyd WD, Vassiliades TA, Karamanoukian HL. Hybrid robotic coronary artery surgery and angioplasty in multivessel coronary artery disease. *Ann. Thorac. Surg.* 2002;74(4):S1358-1362.

[41] Lewis BS, Porat E, Halon DA, Ammar R, Flugelman MY, Khader N, Merdler A, Weisz G, Uretzky G. Same-day combined coronary angioplasty and minimally invasive coronary surgery. *Am. J. Cardiol.* 1999;84(10):1246-1247, A1248.

[42] Wittwer T, Cremer J, Klima U, Wahlers T, Haverich A. Myocardial "hybrid" revascularization: intermediate results of an alternative approach to multivessel coronary artery disease. *J. Thorac. Cardiovasc. Surg.* 1999;118(4):766-767.

[43] Riess FC, Bader R, Kremer P, Kuhn C, Kormann J, Mathey D, Moshar S, Tuebler T, Bleese N, Schofer J. Coronary hybrid revascularization from January 1997 to January 2001: a clinical follow-up. *Ann. Thorac. Surg.* 2002;73(6):1849-1855.

[44] Zenati M, Cohen HA, Griffith BP. Alternative approach to multivessel coronary disease with integrated coronary revascularization. *J. Thorac. Cardiovasc. Surg.* 1999;117(3):439-444; discussion 444-436.

[45] Us MH, Basaran M, Yilmaz M, Yaymaci B, Ulusoy E, Sanioglu S, Ozbek C, Arslan Y, Pocan S, Yilmaz AT. Hybrid coronary revascularization in high-risk patients. *Tex. Heart. Inst. J.* 2006;33(4):458-462.

[46] Gilard M, Bezon E, Cornily JC, Mansourati J, Mondine P, Barra JA, Boschat J. Same-day combined percutaneous coronary intervention and coronary artery surgery. *Cardiology.* 2007;108(4):363-367.

[47] Kon ZN, Brown EN, Tran R, Joshi A, Reicher B, Grant MC, Kallam S, Burris N, Connerney I, Zimrin D, Poston RS. Simultaneous hybrid coronary revascularization reduces postoperative morbidity compared with results from conventional off-pump coronary artery bypass. *J. Thorac. Cardiovasc. Surg.* 2008;135(2):367-375.

[48] Lee MS, Wilentz JR, Makkar RR, Singh V, Nero T, Swistel D, Belsey SJ, Simon C, Rametta S, DeRose J. Hybrid revascularization using percutaneous coronary intervention and robotically assisted minimally invasive direct coronary artery bypass surgery. *J. Invasive. Cardiol.* 2004;16(8):419-425.

[49] Davidavicius G, Van Praet F, Mansour S, Casselman F, Bartunek J, Degrieck I, Wellens F, De Geest R, Vanermen H, Wijns W, De Bruyne B. Hybrid revascularization strategy: a pilot study on the association of robotically enhanced minimally invasive direct coronary artery bypass surgery and fractional-flow-reserve-guided percutaneous coronary intervention. *Circulation.* 2005;112(9 Suppl):I317-322.

[50] Kiaii B, McClure RS, Kostuk WJ, Rayman R, Swinamer S, Dobkowski WB, Novick RJ. Concurrent robotic hybrid revascularization using an enhanced operative suite. *Chest.* 2005;128(6):4046-4048.

[51] Katz MR, Van Praet F, de Canniere D, Murphy D, Siwek L, Seshadri-Kreaden U, Friedrich G, Bonatti J. Integrated coronary revascularization: percutaneous coronary intervention plus robotic totally endoscopic coronary artery bypass. *Circulation.* 2006;114(1 Suppl):I473-476.

[52] Vassiliades TA, Jr., Douglas JS, Morris DC, Block PC, Ghazzal Z, Rab ST, Cates CU. Integrated coronary revascularization with drug-eluting stents: immediate and seven-month outcome. *J. Thorac. Cardiovasc. Surg.* 2006;131(5):956-962.

[53] Bonatti J, Schachner T, Bonaros N, Jonetzko P, Ohlinger A, Ruetzler E, Kolbitsch C, Feuchtner G, Laufer G, Pachinger O, Friedrich G. Simultaneous Hybrid COronary Revascularization Using Totally Endoscopic Left Internal Mammary Artery Bypass Grafting and Placement of RapamycIN Eluting Stents in the SAme IntervenTIONal Session. The COMBINATION Pilot Study. *Cardiology.* 2007;110(2):92-95.

[54] Lloyd CT, Calafiore AM, Wilde P, Ascione R, Paloscia L, Monk CR, Angelini GD. Integrated left anterior small thoracotomy and angioplasty for coronary artery revascularization. *Ann. Thorac. Surg.* 1999;68(3):908-911; discussion 911-902.

[55] Goldstein JA, Safian RD, Aliabadi D, O'Neill WW, Shannon FL, Bassett J, Sakwa M. Intraoperative angiography to assess graft patency after minimally invasive coronary bypass. *Ann. Thorac. Surg.* 1998;66(6):1978-1982.

[56] Byrne JG, Leacche M, Unic D, Rawn JD, Simon DI, Rogers CD, Cohn LH. Staged initial percutaneous coronary intervention followed by valve surgery ("hybrid approach") for patients with complex coronary and valve disease. *J. Am. Coll. Cardiol.* 2005;45(1):14-18.

[57] Gurbel PA, Bliden KP, Hiatt BL, O'Connor CM. Clopidogrel for coronary stenting: response variability, drug resistance, and the effect of pretreatment platelet reactivity. *Circulation.* 2003;107(23):2908-2913.

[58] Weerasinghe A, Taylor KM. The platelet in cardiopulmonary bypass. *Ann. Thorac. Surg.* 1998;66(6):2145-2152.

[59] McCullough PA, Wolyn R, Rocher LL, Levin RN, O'Neill WW. Acute renal failure after coronary intervention: incidence, risk factors, and relationship to mortality. *Am. J. Med.* 1997;103(5):368-375.
[60] Parfrey PS, Griffiths SM, Barrett BJ, Paul MD, Genge M, Withers J, Farid N, McManamon PJ. Contrast material-induced renal failure in patients with diabetes mellitus, renal insufficiency, or both. A prospective controlled study. *N. Engl. J. Med.* 1989;320(3):143-149.
[61] Gleeson TG, Bulugahapitiya S. Contrast-induced nephropathy. *AJR Am. J. Roentgenol.* 2004;183(6):1673-1689.
[62] Rihal CS, Textor SC, Grill DE, Berger PB, Ting HH, Best PJ, Singh M, Bell MR, Barsness GW, Mathew V, Garratt KN, Holmes DR, Jr. Incidence and prognostic importance of acute renal failure after percutaneous coronary intervention. *Circulation.* 2002;105(19):2259-2264.
[63] Hogan JC, Lewis MJ, Henderson AH. N-acetylcysteine fails to attenuate haemodynamic tolerance to glyceryl trinitrate in healthy volunteers. *Br. J. Clin. Pharmacol.* 1989;28(4):421-426.
[64] Mueller C, Buerkle G, Buettner HJ, Petersen J, Perruchoud AP, Eriksson U, Marsch S, Roskamm H. Prevention of contrast media-associated nephropathy: randomized comparison of 2 hydration regimens in 1620 patients undergoing coronary angioplasty. *Arch. Intern. Med.* 2002;162(3):329-336.
[65] Lawlor DK, Moist L, DeRose G, Harris KA, Lovell MB, Kribs SW, Elliot J, Forbes TL. Prevention of contrast-induced nephropathy in vascular surgery patients. *Ann. Vasc. Surg.* 2007;21(5):593-597.
[66] Chen SL, Zhang J, Yei F, Zhu Z, Liu Z, Lin S, Chu J, Yan J, Zhang R, Kwan TW. Clinical outcomes of contrast-induced nephropathy in patients undergoing percutaneous coronary intervention: a prospective, multicenter, randomized study to analyze the effect of hydration and acetylcysteine. *Int. J. Cardiol.* 2008;126(3):407-413.
[67] Schachner T, Bonatti J, Bonaros N, Poeltl R, Feuchtner G, Laufer G, Pachinger O, Friedrich G. Risk factors of postoperative nephropathy in patients undergoing innovative CABG and intraoperative graft angiography. *Eur. J. Cardiothorac. Surg.* 2006;30(3):431-435.
[68] Anesthesiologists ASo. *Guidelines for Nonoperating Room Anesthetizing Locations.* 1994.
[69] Frenzel JC. Anesthesia for the Patient in Remote Diagnostic and Therapeutic Locations. In: Shaw AD, Riedel BJ, Burton AW, Fields AI, Feeley TW, eds. *Acute Care of the Cancer Patient.* New York: Taylor and Francis; 2005:499-504.
[70] Snyder-Ramos SA, Mohnle P, Weng YS, Bottiger BW, Kulier A, Levin J, Mangano DT. The ongoing variability in blood transfusion practices in cardiac surgery. *Transfusion.* 2008;48(7):1284-1299.
[71] Zhao DX, Leacche M, Balaguer JM, Boudoulas KD, Damp JA, Greelish JP, Byrne JG; Writing Group of the Cardiac Surgery, Cardiac Anesthesiology, and Interventional Cardiology Groups at the Vanderbilt Heart and Vascular Institute, Ahmad RM, Ball SK, Cleator JH, Deegan RJ, Eagle SS, Fong PP, Fredi JL, Hoff SJ, Jennings HS 3rd, McPherson JA, Piana RN, Pretorius M, Robbins MA, Slosky DA, Thompson A. *J Am Coll Cardiol.* 2009 Jan 20;53(3):232-41.

In: New Developments in Angiography Research
Editors: K. I. Sanders and A. M. Jackson

ISBN: 978-1-62081-492-5

Chapter VII

A FOLLOW-UP OF IMAGE REGISTRATION TECHNIQUES FOR APPLICATION IN DIGITAL SUBTRACTION ANGIOGRAPHY

Y. Bentoutou[1,*] and N. Taleb[2]
[1]National Center of Space Technology (CNTS),
Arzew, Algeria
[2]Department of Electronics, University of Djillali Liabes,
Sidi Bel Abbes, Algeria

ABSTRACT

Image registration is one of the most important image processing operations in Digital Subtraction Angiography (DSA). In this application, it is necessary to register multiple images of the same sequence in order to reduce patient motion artifacts. The registered images are then subtracted in order to evaluate the progress of a disease and/or a treatment procedure. In this chapter, a follow-up of some recent automatic registration techniques for digital X-ray angiography images is presented. A first method is based on a 3-D space-time motion evaluation and on an edge-detection approach leading to the selection of a set of control points from which pixels having their values changed due to motion are separated from those due to contrast flow, by means of detecting the peak iodine opacification. A second technique is based on local similarity detection by means of template matching according to the combined invariants-based similarity measure. The main characteristic of the third approach is that it combines the two previous ones to establish correspondences between the potentially matched movement points detected from the two images. The results clearly indicate that the third registration algorithm is much better able to recover patient motion than the other ones and would therefore be the method of choice for automatic registration of angiographic images.

Keywords: Image registration; Template matching; Thin Plate Spline; Motion correction; Digital subtraction angiography; Medical imaging

---

* E-mail: bentyou@univ-sba.dz.

1. INTRODUCTION

1.1. Motivation

In modern medicine, Digital Subtraction Angiography (DSA) is a powerful technique for the visualization of blood vessels in a sequence of X-ray images [1-12]. In this technique, a sequence of two-dimensional (2-D) digital X-ray projection images is taken to show the passage of the injected contrast material through the patient's vessels of interest. The first few images in the sequence do not have any information about the blood flow, since the contrast agent would not have passed through the vessels yet. These images are usually called mask images. The images of the sequence obtained during the passage of the contrast material through the vessels of interest are often referred to as contrast images or live images.

In ordinary X-ray projection images, blood vessels are hardly visible. This may introduce a reduction in the amount of diagnostic information that can be extracted from the images. Subtraction of the mask image from a contrast image is the simplest form of temporal filtering in DSA and is the way to obtain visible vessels. It is based on the assumption that the background structures of the contrast images are exactly aligned, and have equal gray-level distributions. However, this is not a valid assumption when dealing with angiographic image sequences, mainly because of two reasons.

- Patient motion that causes the subtraction images to show artifacts may reduce the diagnostic value of DSA images.
- Images taken at different time instances will always differ in some respect, due to fluctuations in the power of the X-ray source or noise in the image intensifier and the subsequent imaging chain.

1.2. Present State of the Art

The major problem encountered in DSA images is the presence of motion artifacts, which arise from the misalignment of successive images in the sequence. Such artifacts can lead to misdiagnosis or rejection of a DSA image sequence. In the latter case, the patient would have to retake the examination, which is invasive because it requires X-ray exposure, injection of contrast material, and venous, arterial, or ventricular catheterization. In order to overcome this problem and to improve the diagnostic value of DSA images, special precautions concerning the patient and the acquisition system were taken to prevent patient motion. However, in many cases, artifacts cannot be entirely avoided and one is forced to resort to image registration techniques. The purpose of image registration (or matching) is to spatially align two or more images taken at different times.

Most image registration algorithms work correctly when the compared misregistered images are very similar but frequently lead to misregistration when dissimilarities are present in the images (i.e., angiographic images acquired by a nonideal DSA system are usually corrupted by spatial degradations like blur and additive noise).

Current clinical DSA imaging systems are equipped with a so-called pixel shifting technique. This technique is easy to implement [3,13] and is based on the assumption that artifacts are caused by gross translational motion only. Several clinical evaluations following the introduction of DSA in the early eighties revealed that this assumption is not valid for a substantial number of examinations. In most cases, patient motion is more complex and cannot be modeled by such a basic transformation. In this situation, a correction in one part of the image implies the introduction of new artifacts in other parts [11].

In order to be able to correct for more complex patient motion, several techniques have been proposed, including template matching [14-27] and three-dimensional (3-D) linear prediction techniques [28]. However, most of these techniques have not led to algorithms that are sufficiently fast so as to be acceptable for integration in clinical applications [27].

In order to be able to correct for more complex patient motion, registration techniques should be designed so as to have more local control.

1.3. Registration Techniques

General overviews of image registration techniques have been given by Maintz and Viergever [29], Meijering et al. [30], and Zitova and Flusser [31]. A great variety of registration methods use a limited set of corresponding control points or landmarks to define the geometrical transformation [29-31]. Rigid and affine registration methods can only cope with global differences, for example, translation, rotation, and scaling. In many cases, however elastic or non rigid methods are required to cope with local differences between the images.

The point-based registration process is usually carried out in four steps. The first step consists of selection of a set of features on one image. Next, each feature in one image is compared with potential corresponding features in the other image. Features with similar attributes are accepted as matches and are called control points (CP). After the CP sets have been matched, the parameters of the best geometrical transformation, which models the deformation between the images, are estimated. Finally, the transformation is executed.

An efficient approach of image registration applied to digital angiography and suitable for clinical use must satisfy the following constraints:

a) The registration procedure must be accurate and fully automated.
b) The patient motion and the gray-level variations in the contrast images which are usually corrupted by spatial degradations, blurring, and random noise must both be corrected globally and locally.
c) The selected window used for the calculations of the registration parameters must be allowed to contain in part the vascular structures, which have to be corrected.
d) The registration approach must be elastic or non-rigid in order to cope with local residual artifacts.
e) The algorithms must be computationally cheap and relatively fast in order to be implemented on DSA systems for a routine use.

Several image registration techniques have been developed [29-31]. Unfortunately, none of these techniques has been shown to satisfy all of the above constraints. For point-based techniques, identical control points have to be identified manually, which is either time-consuming for an operator or requires the prior attachment of markers. In both cases the accuracy is not guaranteed. Image registration with the most developed class of intensity-based techniques works correctly when the compared misregistered images are very similar but frequently lead to misregistration when dissimilarities are present in the images (i.e., angiographic images acquired by a nonideal DSA system are usually corrupted by spatial degradations like blur and additive noise). In this case, these methods do not satisfy constraints (b) and (c).

1.4. The Aim of the Chapter

Recently, three new, fast, and accurate fully automatic registration techniques were developed [12, 32-34]. The first method is based on a 3D space-time motion evaluation for separating pixels changing values because of motion from those changing values because of contrast flow. It is capable of aligning pairs of angiographic images within few seconds [12]. The second one is based on an image content driven control point selection mechanism and on modern graphics hardware for image warping [32].

The algorithm was clinically evaluated on cerebral DSA images and it was found to result in better image quality and to be considerably less time consuming [32]. The third method combines the first two developed methods in order to improve the registration quality. In this technique, the 3D space-time motion detection algorithm is used for extracting movement points with accuracy. It is based on template matching according to the combined invariants-based similarity measure for movement point displacement computation [33,34].

The purpose of this chapter is to present a follow-up of the three newly proposed automatic registration techniques for patient motion correction in digital angiographic images and to compare these automatic methods with the standard manual technique used on DSA systems.

The designed algorithms have the capability to register images both globally and locally, even when applied to the worst DSA cases. These algorithms, introducing local processing on areas of interest consisting of movement pixels only, are computationally efficient, and as will be seen, demonstrate the capability to remove all motion changes when applied to real coronary arteries.

The rest of the chapter is organized as follows. The 3-D space-time motion evaluation approach is described in section 2. Section 3 describes the second image registration method based on the combined invariants. Section 4 describes the combination of these two proposed registration approaches. Results of experiments on clinical data sets are reported in section 5. Finally, the related conclusions are given in section 6.

2. Method 1: A Fast Method for Motion ArtifactsRemoval

This method is based on a 3-d space-time motion evaluation for removing patient motion artifacts from DSA images. It involves the extraction of the opacified vessels from the background anatomy by an 'a priori' knowledge of the probable variation of arterial iodine concentration with time following an intravenous injection of contrast material.

Figure 1 shows the iodine concentration as a function of time. The resulting curve represents the signal, which, in this work, is to be isolated and is called the contrast dilution curve. It is characterized by a significant rise followed by a significant fall in the iodine concentration. Figures 2 and 3 show the gray-level variations in two different regions of interest for two sets of digital angiographic images acquired during the flow of contrast material through an area of interest. The first region contains contrasted vessels.

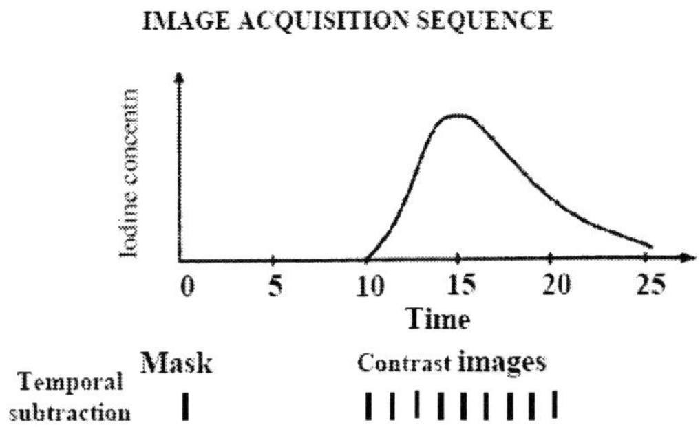

Figure 1. Image acquisition sequence for temporal subtraction.

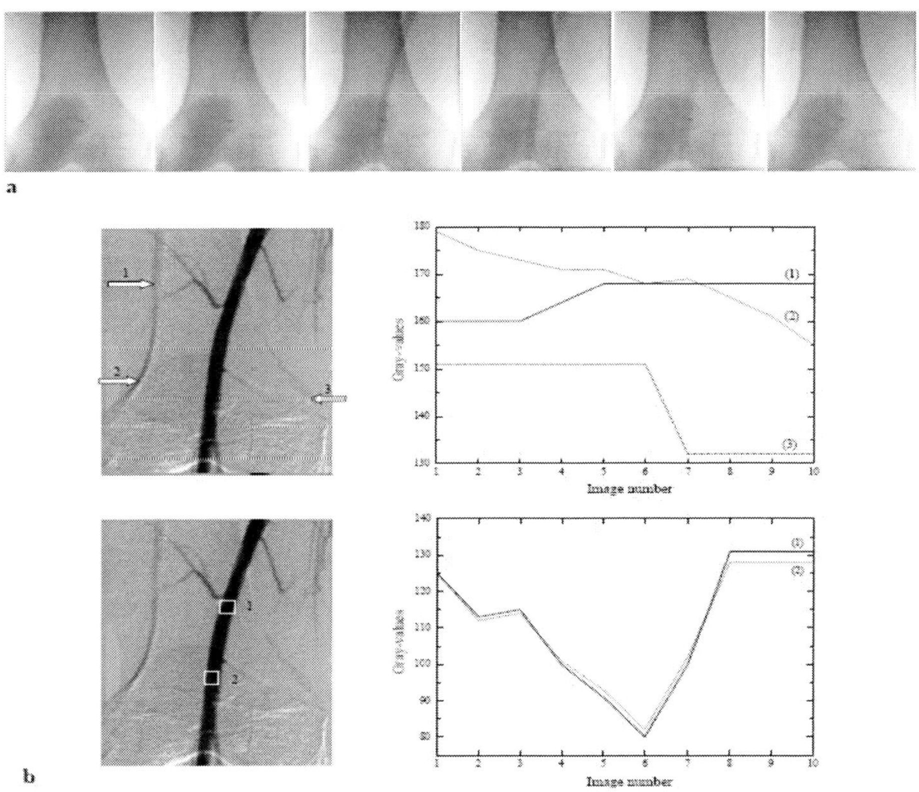

Figure 2. (a) First digital angiographic image sequence (some images of the sequence: top left to right then bottom left to right) used in the experiments and showing the passage of the injected contrast material through the vessels of interest. (b) The gray-level variations in different regions of interest. Left-Column: Regions containing strong object edges (indicated by white arrows) and contrasted vessels (indicated by white boxes). Right-Column: the corresponding gray-level variations.

The second region contains strong object edges because in DSA images artifacts can only occur at image edges. From these figures it can be seen that the resulting curves for the first region (containing contrasted vessels) contain only one peak, which is characterized by a significant fall followed by a significant rise in the gray-level. This peak corresponds to the peak iodine opacification that occurs in an image located at around the middle of the sequence. In this case, the sixth image is taken at the time of maximum opacification. The intensity associated with all pixels belonging to contrasted vessels varies rapidly in time resulting in only one peak. In the case of the second region (containing strong object edges), such a peak is not guaranteed to exist. In most cases, the intensity associated with all pixels belonging to image edges varies slowly in time from one level to another [11, 28].

These two observations imply that the motion artifacts can be removed from the contrast images in the sequence by isolating the opacified vessels. This is done by extracting all pixels having their values changed rapidly in time and resulting in only one peak (pixels belonging to opacified vessels) from the unwanted information (background structures). This peak is defined as a sample that is greater than both its predecessors and its successors.

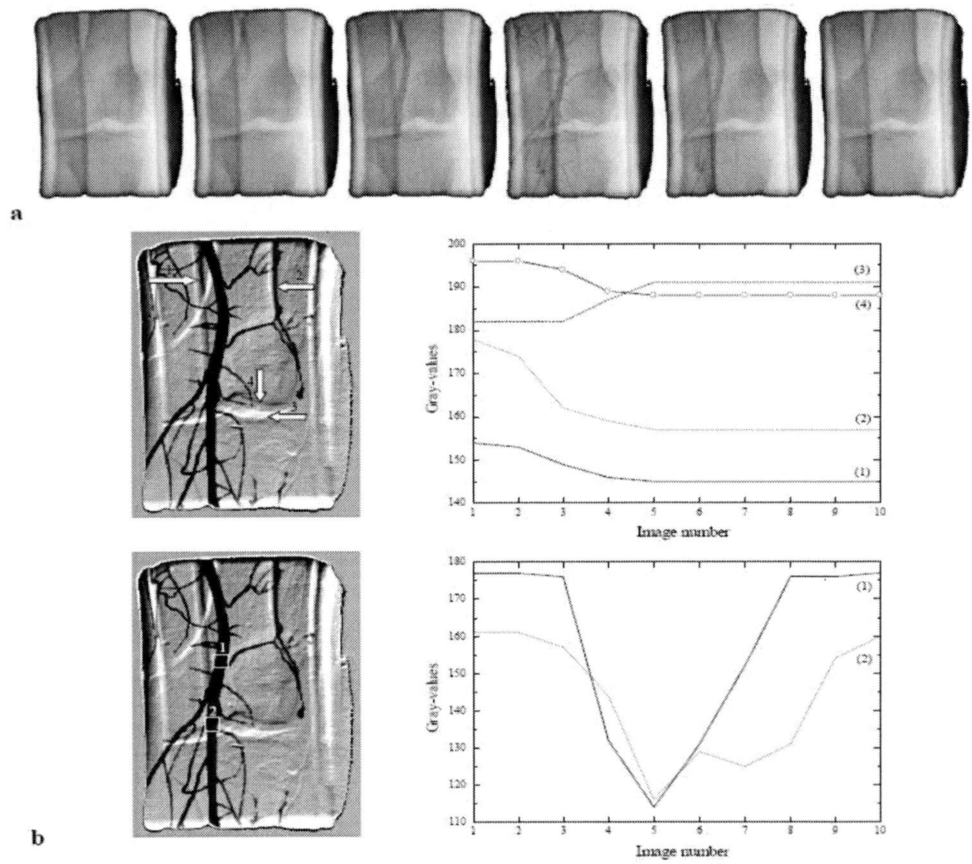

Figure 3. (a) Second digital angiographic image sequence (some images of the sequence: top left to right then bottom left to right) used in the experiments and showing the passage of the injected contrast material through the vessels of interest. (b) The gray-level variations in different regions of interest. *Left-Column:* Regions containing strong object edges (indicated by white arrows) and contrasted vessels (indicated by white boxes). *Right-Column***:** the corresponding gray-level variations.

2.1. Control Points Selection

In order to correct for motion artifacts and gray-level distortions, a possible approach is to process all pixels belonging to the image. However, this is computationally expensive. It has to be noted that in the particular case of DSA images, artifacts only appear in those regions where strong object edges are present in the unsubtracted images. Clearly misalignment between mask and contrast images can only occur at the image edges, and therefore one easy way to speed up the algorithm and to reduce the computation time to a clinically acceptable level is to process pixels belonging to image edges only (referred to as the control points), instead of processing all image pixels. Obviously, the less complex is the image, the faster is the algorithm [11].

In this implementation, the edge-detection approach has two advantages: (1) The computation time is reduced with respect to taking all image pixels; (2) The control points are chosen at these positions where the artifacts can be expected to be the largest.

The first step in the design of the proposed algorithm consists of finding the image edges. The image to be processed for edges is first sharpened using high-emphasis filtering [35]. The gradient image and the edge-direction map are then computed using the Sobel operator. Combining the gradient image with the edge-direction map and the threshold map, and applying a local connectivity algorithm [36] will permit the derivation of a better edge map image. An example of control point selection based on this approach is shown in Figure 4.

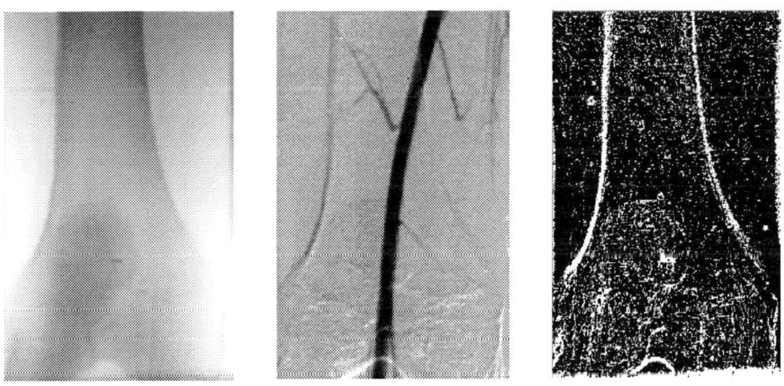

Figure 4. Control points selection. (a) Mask image of the first 512 × 512 × 10 digital angiographic image sequence. (b) Subtraction of the mask image from a contrast image, showing considerable bone-tissue misregistration. (c) Edge image obtained from the mask image, showing the set of control points (white dots).

2.2. Motion Artifacts Removal

A digital 2-D discrete image sequence can be thought of as a 3-D space–time signal $I(i,j,n)$ of size $M \times M \times N$ with values representing the pixel intensity. The spatial variables are i and j, while n is the time variable.

The single subtraction of the mask image $I(i,j,0)$ from one of the contrast images $I(i,j,n)$, $n \in [1,N-1] \subset \mathbf{N}$, can be written as

$$d_n(i,j)=I(i,j,n)-I(i,j,0) \tag{1}$$

Consider that for a pixel p_{ij} at position (i,j) in the mask image, the vector $\overline{a}_{ij}$ that consists of the pixel values for each image in the sequence $\{ I(i,j,n) \}, n\in[0,N-1]\subset \mathbf{N}$ is given by

$$\overline{a}_{ij}=[I(i,j,0)I(i,j,1)....I(i,j,N)] \tag{2}$$

Notice first that neither the first nor the last few elements of $\overline{a}_{ij}$ can be a peak (the first and the last few images in the sequences do not have much information about the blood flow). For that reason, the detection of peaks can be applied to the contrasted images chosen near the time of maximum opacification. The number of these images depends on the total number of images in the sequence. A typical number is 5 images for a sequence of 10 to 14 images.

Let $\Pi(\overline{a}_{ij})$ denote the peak element of $\overline{a}_{ij}$. This peak is defined as the minimal element of $\overline{a}_{ij}$ that satisfies the following constraints:

a) This minimal element is smaller than both its predecessors and its successors.
b) This element cannot be the first or the last element of $\overline{a}_{ij}$.

$$\Pi(\overline{a}_{ij})=min(\overline{a}_{ij})=I(i,j,k) \tag{3}$$

where $k\in[m-L,m+L]$ is the time index of the minimal element, *m* the time of maximum opacification, and *L* defines the allowable interval of minimal elements around *m*. Notice that this peak occurs at an image located around the middle of the sequence (i.e., one of the images $I(i,j,m-L)$, $I(i,j,m-L+1)$ to $I(i,j,m+L)$) which is not the case for a pixel changing value due to motion. For any peak element detected outside this range of images, the corresponding pixel will be considered as a pixel belonging to background anatomy, otherwise this pixel belongs to a contrasted vessel, having its value varying because of the contrast flow. Thus this pixel will be separated from pixels belonging to background anatomy (having their values changing because of motion).

2.3. Algorithm 1

Given an image sequence of size *M*×*M*×*N*, the cancellation of motion artifacts by means of blood vessels detection in a digital angiographic image sequence is accomplished by carrying out the following steps:

1) Sharpen the mask image. It is based on high-emphasis filtering with the application of a digital Laplacian to the image [35].

2) Compute the gradient image and the edge-direction map. The gradient image and its orientation map are computed using the Sobel operator. The final edge image is acquired after applying some local connectivity information [36] to the gradient image, in combination with the edge-direction map and the threshold map.
3) Create a scratch image $s(i,j)$ where all pixels have some identical and particular values that are not attributed to real images; a simple example is pixels having all the same negative value "-1".
4) For each control point p_{ij} (pixel having the value "1", i.e., pixel belonging to an edge) at position (i,j) in the edge map image, compute vector $\overline{a}_{ij}$.
   - Detect the minimal element of $\overline{a}_{ij}$ according to Eq. (3).
   - If this element satisfies conditions (*a*) and (*b*) then; control point p_{ij} belongs to a contrasted vessel, and its value is plugged into the scratch image at the same position (i,j), i.e., $s(i,j)=I(i,j,m)$, where $I(i,j,m)$ denotes the contrast image of maximum opacification.
   - Else if this element does not satisfy constraints (*a*)-(*b*) then; control point p_{ij} belongs to background anatomy, and in this case, its corresponding value in the mask image is plugged into the scratch image at position (i,j), i.e., $s(i,j)=I(i,j,0)$, where $I(i,j,0)$ denotes the mask image.
5) At the end of step 4, all pixel values that have been changed from the "-1" value in the scratch image are the corrected pixel values in the image of maximum opacification. Thus, these pixel values are plugged into the image of maximum opacification and the result is the corrected contrast image that has the same background anatomy as that of the mask image.
6) Perform the subtraction between the image of maximum opacification and the mask image. This subtraction results in a high-contrast image of the vessels.

3. Method 2: An Invariant Approach for the Registration of Digital Angiographic Images

In this method, the registration process is carried out in three steps. The first step consists of selecting automatically a set of control points $P=\{p_i\}$ from the contrast image. In the second step, the displacements of the selected control points $p_i \in P$ are computed by means of template matching using the combined invariants-based similarity measure.

The new coordinates of the selected control points $p_i \in P$ in the mask image constitute the corresponding set of control points $Q=\{q_i\}$ in this image. Finally, the parameters of the best transformation, which models the deformation between the images, are estimated using the two sets of corresponding control points (P and Q).

The final correction is performed according to this transformation by warping one of the images with respect to the other using the thin- plate spline (TPS) interpolation function [37].

3.1. Control Points Selection

In the particular case of DSA images, artifacts only appear in those regions where strong object edges are present in the unsubtracted images. Clearly, misalignment between mask and contrast images can only occur at the image edges, and therefore one easy way to speed up the algorithm and to reduce the computation time to a clinically acceptable level is to process pixels belonging to image edges only (referred to as the control points), instead of processing all image edges.

Obviously, the less complex is the image, the faster is the algorithm.

In this implementation, the edge-detection approach is applied to the contrast images. This approach is not applied to the mask images, because the boundaries of the vessels would not be detected.

The same argument holds for the application of edge-detection to the subtraction images in the case of gross patient motion. Clearly, these two cases do not present the advantage of point (2) and therefore do not satisfy constraint (b) mentioned in section 1.3.

The first step in the selection of the control points consists of finding image edges. The location of edges can easily be computed by detecting local maxima of the gray-level gradient magnitude. Since edges are scale dependent image features, they can only be detected properly using derivatives calculated at the proper scale.

The commonly used edge detection filter for this purpose is Gaussian derivative, which allows finer tuning to detect the required edge scale [38]. It should be noted that it is necessary to indicate which edges are important for extracting adequate control points. This is done by thresholding the gradient magnitude image at a value Φ, resulting in a binary image in which there are connected regions that are of interest.

The following is a summary of the different steps to be followed in the selection of control points.

1. Compute the gradient magnitude at scale S of the contrast image. It is based on an edge detection filtering with the application of Gaussian derivative [38].
2. Extract potential artifact regions by means of thresholding the gradient magnitude image at level Φ.
3. Choose a moving window W of $w \times w$ pixels that will sweep over all the pixels in the thresholded edge image. The size of this window depends on the size of the images themselves. This window will be used later for the measure of match.
4. Move the above window, line by line, through the thresholded edge image. If a pixel value is "1" (pixel belonging to an edge), then this pixel is considered to be a control point.
5. To avoid taking all pixels belonging to an edge inside the same window as control points, take just one pixel as a control point and, assign a "0" value to all the rest of the pixels in the same window.
6. Repeat steps 4 and 5 until going through all pixels belonging to all edges.

An example of control point selection based on this approach is shown in Figure 5.

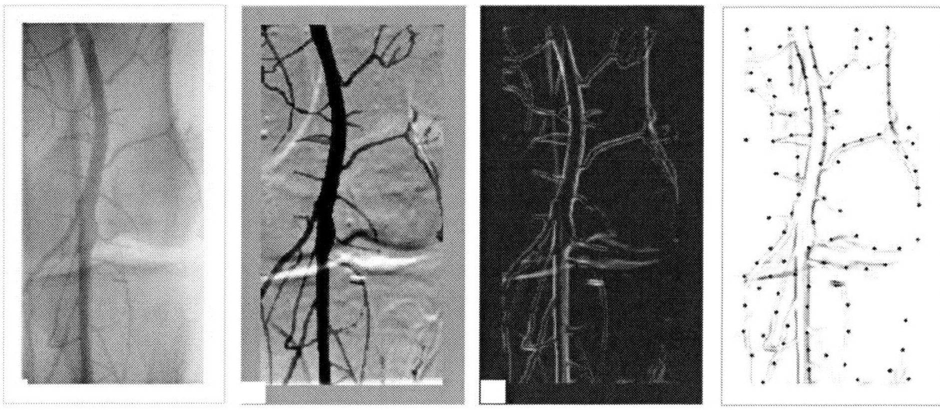

(a) (b) (c) (d)

Figure 5. Control points selection. (a) A contrast image from a 512 × 512 × 10 digital angiographic image sequence. (b) The subtraction of the contrast image from the mask image showing considerable bone-tissue misregistration. (c) Thresholded gradient-magnitude image of the contrast image. (d) The set of selected control points (black dots), with the edge image superimposed.

3.2. Control Points Displacements Computation

Given a two-dimensional discrete image sequence $I(x, y, n)$ of size $M \times M \times N$, techniques for the automatic computation of local motion of certain objects of one of the images, $I(x, y, n_1)$, $n_1 \in [0, N-1] \subset \mathrm{N}$ with respect to a successive image $I(x, y, n_2)$, $n_1 < n_2 < N-1$ in the sequence, can be divided into two categories: (1) optic-flow techniques and (2) template matching based techniques, both of which have distinct advantages [27,30]. The method described here falls into the latter category.

In practice, the basic assumptions of optic-flow techniques do not apply to digital X-ray images [27,30]. Also, these techniques are sensitive to the inflow of contrast. Template matching techniques, however, can be made relatively robust against this phenomenon, by applying an adequate similarity measure.

Template matching techniques are based on the assumption that the displacement d of every pixel in an image $I(x, y, n_1)$ can be approximated by taking a small window W around the pixel and finding the corresponding window in a successive image $I(x, y, n_2)$, $n_2 > n_1$, in the sequence according to a certain similarity measure [30].

3.2.1. Similarity Measures

The most important aspect of template matching is the similarity measure that is used to determine the degree of resemblance of windows in successive frames.

Several measures have been devised and applied to angiographic images, including normalized cross-correlation (NCC) [14,39], the correlation coefficient (CC) [11,39,40], statistical correlation (SC) [41], stochastic and deterministic sign change (SSC and DSC)

[19,42,43], the sum of the absolute values of differences (SAVD) [24,44-46], the mean of the absolute values of the differences (MAVD) [47,48-53], coincident bit counting (CBC) [54,55], the variance of differences (VOD) [20], and the histogram of differences (HOD) [56-59, 21-23]. However, most of these similarity measures do not satisfy the four constraints that have been emphasized in the introduction of this chapter.

They are sensitive to mean gray-level offsets and local dissimilarities caused by contrasted vessels [27]. In addition to these fundamental problems, there are other factors that may complicate the process of finding the optimal correspondence between successive images. These are due to imperfections of the acquisition system, such as limited spatial resolution, gray-level quantization, blur, noise or the effects of time-varying scatter.

Measures that are very robust against this phenomenon are those that are based on the moment-based combined invariants (i.e., invariants with respect to degradations composed from symmetric blur and another geometric or gray-level transform) [60]. Detailed definitions of these combined invariants can be found in literature (see [60]).

The moments $m_{pq}^{(I)}$ of a binary image $I(i,j)$ are given by

$$m_{pq}^{(I)} = \sum_{i=1}^{N}\sum_{j=1}^{N} i^p \, j^q \, I(i,j) \tag{4}$$

where $(p+q)$ is the order of moment and $(N \times N)$ is the size of the image.

The central moments $\mu_{pq}^{(I)}$ of order $(p+q)$ of the image $I(i,j)$ are defined as

$$\mu_{pq}^{(I)} = \sum_{i=1}^{N}\sum_{j=1}^{N} \left(i - x_t^{(I)}\right)^p \left(j - y_t^{(I)}\right)^q I(i,j) \tag{5}$$

where the coordinates $x_t^{(I)} = \dfrac{m_{10}^{(I)}}{m_{00}^{(I)}}$ and $y_t^{(I)} = \dfrac{m_{01}^{(I)}}{m_{00}^{(I)}}$ denote the centroid of $I(i,j)$.

The combined invariants (features based on image moments and invariant to symmetric blur, change of contrast and translation) used in this research, are given by the following equation:

$$C'(p,q)^{(I)} = \begin{cases} \dfrac{\mu_{pq}^{(I)}}{\mu_{00}^{(I)}} - \dfrac{1}{\mu_{00}^{(I)}} \displaystyle\sum_{n=0}^{p}\sum_{m=0}^{q} \binom{p}{n}\binom{q}{m} C'(p-n, q-m)^{(I)} . \mu_{nm}^{(I)} & \text{if } (p+q) \text{ is odd} \\ 0 & \text{if } (p+q) \text{ is even} \end{cases} \tag{6}$$

where $0 < n+m < p+q$. The number $r = p+q$ is called the order of the combined invariant.

In this chapter, the set of combined invariants of the third and fifth orders is used. It was shown [60] that these combined invariants are sufficiently robust with respect to noise.

The local displacement for a structure in the mask image can be estimated by defining a certain window W of $w \times w$ pixels containing this structure, and by finding the corresponding window in a contrast image in the sequence by means of combined invariants-based similarity measure.

For this measure, the distance between two windows W_1 and W_2 is defined as

$$d_r(w_1, w_2) = \left\| \vec{C}(r)^{(w_1)} - \vec{C}(r)^{(w_2)} \right\| \tag{7}$$

where $\|.\|$ is Euclidean norm in $l_2(k_r)$ space (k_r is the size of $\vec{C}(r)$), and the vector $\vec{C}(r)$ of combined invariants is defined as

$$\vec{C}(r) = \left(\overline{C}_3, \overline{C}_5, \ldots, \overline{C}_r\right) \tag{8}$$

where r is the order of the combined invariant, and the vector $\overline{C}_r$ is defined as

$$\overline{C}_r = \left(C'(0,r), C'(1,r-1), \ldots, C'(r,0)\right) \tag{9}$$

In the case of optimal alignment, the distance between the two windows is nil ($d_r = 0$).

With this similarity measure, the size of the windows is not determined by the dimensions of the region of interest, but rather by the minimum amount of information required to obtain reliable estimates for the displacement of the corresponding control points. This in turn highly depends on the criterion, which is employed to determine similarity and may also depend on image content. It was shown in that an adequate window size of 21×21 pixels yields a good compromise between computational speed and statistical reliability [32].

The displacements of control points are determined by carrying out the following steps:

1. For every control point, choose a moving window W_1 of $w \times w$ pixels around this point in the contrast image.
2. Assuming that misregistration parameters would not exceed a "5" degree angle for image rotation and a "10" pixel shift for image translation (reasonable practical assumptions), rotate this window by an angle of "-5" degrees and calculate the combined invariants vectors $\vec{C}(r)^{(W_1)}$ and $\vec{C}(r)^{(W_2)}$ of W_1 and the corresponding non-rotated window W_2 in the mask image, respectively.
3. Calculate the distance d_r between these two windows in the invariant space, taking into consideration the amount of the maximum translational shift. Save the translational shift giving the minimum distance.
4. Repeat steps 2,3, and 4 after each rotation of a "+1" degree angle of the preceding window (W_1) until reaching a rotation angle of "+5" degrees. After each rotation, keep saving the translational shift according to minimum distance in the invariant

space. At the end, the values of the translational shifts will correspond to the displacements of control points up to integer precision.

3.2.2. Subpixel Precision

Meijering et al. [27] indicated that even subpixel misalignments may produce significant artifacts in the subtraction images. Therefore, it is necessary to provide means to obtain subpixel precision in the displacements computation because the described matching approach only determines the displacements up to integer precision. Since the image pixels constitute the only available information about the represented scene, this inevitably requires some form of interpolation.

In order to obtain subpixel accuracy in the displacements computation, several approaches have been proposed, such as analytical match-interpolation methods [20,30] and image-interpolation methods [27,44].

In the image interpolation approach, subpixel accuracy can be achieved by translating the mask image by subpixel increments in the local region around the initial best match position [44]. This method is computationally very expensive compared to the analytical match-interpolation methods. An analytical match-interpolation method [20] is used in this chapter. In this method, subpixel accuracy is achieved by interpolating in the match measure surface to estimate the position of the peak. Separate horizontal and vertical quadratic interpolation is used to refine the estimates of the two components of each movement point p_i.

Given the discrete match measure surface $M(x, y)$ and the best match position (x_0, y_0), the estimated continuous coordinates (x', y') of the match peak are calculated as

$$x' = x_0 - \frac{1}{2} + \frac{M(x_0, y_0) - M(x_0 - 1, y_0)}{2M(x_0, y_0) - M(x_0 - 1, y_0) - M(x_0 + 1, y_0)}$$
$$y' = y_0 - \frac{1}{2} + \frac{M(x_0, y_0) - M(x_0, y_0 - 1)}{2M(x_0, y_0) - M(x_0, y_0 - 1) - M(x_0, y_0 + 1)} \quad (10)$$

The exact coordinates (x_i', y_i'), in the mask image of each movement point $p_i = (x_i, y_i)$, $i = 1, 2, \ldots m$, constitute the second set of movement points $Q = \{q_i\}$ with $q_i = (x_i', y_i')$, $i = 1, 2, \ldots m$.

3.3. Image Warping

Given the two sets of corresponding control points, $P = \{p_i\}$ and $Q = \{q_i\}$, the correction is performed by warping the mask image. We performed mask image warping by applying elastic thin-plate spline (TPS) interpolation function [37] on the two sets of control points. The thin-plate splines are interpolating functions, representing the distortion at each control point exactly, and defining a minimum-curvature surface between control points. It is a flexible transformation that allows rotation, translation, scaling, and skewing. It also allows lines to bend according to the thin-plate spline model. Therefore, a large number of deformations can be characterized by the thin-plate spline model.

The thin-plate spline interpolation function can be written as

$$\mathbf{h}(\mathbf{x}) = A\mathbf{x} + \boldsymbol{t} + \sum_{i=1}^{m} \mathbf{W}_i \boldsymbol{K}\left(\|\mathbf{x} - \mathbf{x}_i\|\right) \tag{11}$$

where A, $\boldsymbol{t}$ are the affine transformation parameters matrices, $\mathbf{W}_i$ are the weights of the non-linear radial interpolation function $\boldsymbol{K}$, and $\mathbf{x}_i$ are the control points. The function $\boldsymbol{K}(r)$ is the solution of the biharmonic equation ($\Delta^2 \boldsymbol{K} = 0$) that satisfies the condition of bending energy minimization, namely $\boldsymbol{K}(r) = r^2 \log(r^2)$. To solve for the x, y components, the transformation $\mathbf{h}$ is defined from two sets of m corresponding control point pairs as:

$$\begin{aligned} x' &= h_x(x,y) = a_{11}x + a_{12}y + t_x + \sum_{i=1}^{m} W_{xi} \boldsymbol{K}\left(\|(x_i, y_i) - (x,y)\|\right) \\ y' &= h_y(x,y) = a_{21}x + a_{22}y + t_y + \sum_{i=1}^{m} W_{yi} \boldsymbol{K}\left(\|(x_i, y_i) - (x,y)\|\right) \end{aligned} \tag{12}$$

with parameters a_{11}, a_{12}, a_{21}, a_{22}, t_x, and t_y representing the linear affine transformation, and with parameters W_{xi} and W_{yi} representing the weights of the function $\boldsymbol{K}$.

The warping of the mask image with respect to the contrast image is accomplished by carrying out the following steps:

1. Given the two sets P and Q of m corresponding control point pairs, the parameters of the affine transformation A and $\boldsymbol{t}$ are obtained using the following equation:

$$\mathbf{y} = \mathbf{Mz} \tag{13}$$

where

$$\boldsymbol{y} = \begin{bmatrix} x'_1 \\ y'_1 \\ x'_2 \\ y'_2 \\ \vdots \\ x'_m \\ y'_m \end{bmatrix},$$

$$\mathbf{M} = \begin{bmatrix} x_1 & y_1 & 0 & 0 & 1 & 0 \\ 0 & 0 & x_1 & y_1 & 0 & 1 \\ x_2 & y_2 & 0 & 0 & 1 & 0 \\ 0 & 0 & x_2 & y_2 & 0 & 1 \\ \vdots & \vdots & \vdots & \vdots & \vdots & \vdots \\ x_m & y_m & 0 & 0 & 1 & 0 \\ 0 & 0 & x_m & y_m & 0 & 1 \end{bmatrix},$$

and

$$\mathbf{z} = \begin{bmatrix} a_{11} \\ a_{12} \\ a_{21} \\ a_{22} \\ t_x \\ t_y \end{bmatrix}$$

$a_{11}, a_{12}, a_{21}, a_{22}, t_x$, and t_y are the affine transformation parameters and found by taking the pseudo inverse of the matrix $\mathbf{M}$.

$$\mathbf{z} = \left(\mathbf{M}^{\mathrm{T}}\mathbf{M}\right)^{-1}\left(\mathbf{M}^{\mathrm{T}}\mathbf{y}\right) \tag{14}$$

where $\mathbf{M}^{\mathrm{T}}$ is the transpose of $\mathbf{M}$ and $\left(\mathbf{M}^{\mathrm{T}}\mathbf{M}\right)^{-1}$ denotes the inverse of $\mathbf{M}^{\mathrm{T}}\mathbf{M}$.

2. The two sets of corresponding control point pairs are then used to calculate the weights W_{xi} and W_{yi} using the equations:

$$\begin{bmatrix} x_1' - a_{11}x_1 - a_{12}y_1 - t_x \\ x_2' - a_{11}x_2 - a_{12}y_2 - t_x \\ \vdots \\ x_m' - a_{11}x_m - a_{12}y_m - t_x \end{bmatrix} = \begin{bmatrix} 0 & K(r_{12}) & \dots & K(r_{1m}) \\ K(r_{21}) & 0 & \dots & K(r_{2m}) \\ \vdots & \vdots & & \vdots \\ K(r_{m1}) & K(r_{m2}) & \dots & 0 \end{bmatrix} \begin{bmatrix} W_{x1} \\ W_{x2} \\ \vdots \\ W_{xm} \end{bmatrix} \tag{15}$$

$$\begin{bmatrix} y_1' - a_{21}x_1 - a_{22}y_1 - t_y \\ y_2' - a_{21}x_2 - a_{22}y_2 - t_y \\ \vdots \\ y_m' - a_{21}x_m - a_{22}y_m - t_y \end{bmatrix} = \begin{bmatrix} 0 & K(r_{12}) & \dots & K(r_{1m}) \\ K(r_{21}) & 0 & \dots & K(r_{2m}) \\ \vdots & \vdots & & \vdots \\ K(r_{m1}) & K(r_{m2}) & \dots & 0 \end{bmatrix} \begin{bmatrix} W_{y1} \\ W_{y2} \\ \vdots \\ W_{ym} \end{bmatrix} \tag{16}$$

where

$$r_{ij} = \left\| (x_i, y_i) - (x'_j, y'_j) \right\|$$

and

$$\boldsymbol{K}(r) = r^2 \log(r^2).$$

3. The complete set of parameters, defining the interpolating registration transformation is then used to transform the mask image values. It should be noted that in order to be able to carry out the warping of the mask image with respect to the contrast image, it is required to have a complete description of the TPS interpolation function (Equation 12). That is, this function must be known for every point in the image. So far, we have only described the method for computing the TPS function of a selected set of control points, under the assumption that the remainder of the field could be obtained by linear interpolation. Detailed algebraic treatment of this TPS based warping can be found in literature (see [37]).

3.4. Algorithm 2

The algorithm here is a summary of the operations involved in the registration of two images of a digital angiographic image sequence, presented and discussed in the previous sections.

Given a two-dimensional discrete image sequence $I(x, y, n)$ of size $M \times M \times N$, the registration of a mask image $I(x, y, 0)$ with respect to one of the contrast images $I(x, y, n)$, $n \in [1, N-1] \subset \mathrm{N}$ is accomplished by carrying out the following steps:

1. Using an edge-detection approach based on Gaussian derivative, select the set of control points $P = \{p_i\}$ in the contrast image $I(x, y, n)$, $n \in [1, N-1] \subset N$ by following steps 1 to 6 of section 3.1.
2. Given the set of control points P, determine the displacement of every selected control point $p_i \in P$ using a template matching technique based on the combined invariants-based similarity measure in a small window of $w \times w$ pixels around the selected control point (steps 1 to 4 of section 3.2).
3. Given the estimated best match position (x_{0i}, y_{0i}) of each control point p_i, determine the coordinates of the best match, (x'_i, y'_i), to subpixel accuracy (Equation (10) of section 3.2.2).
4. Given the two sets P and Q of corresponding control point pairs in the two images, warp the mask image by using the thin-plate spline (TPS) interpolation function on the two sets of control points (steps 1 to 3 of section 3.3).

4. Method 3: 3D Space-Time Motion Detection for an Invariant Image Registration Approach in Digital Subtraction Angiography

In this method, the registration process is carried out in three steps [33,34]. The first step consists of selecting automatically a set of movement points $P = \{(x_i, y_i),\ i = 1,2,..., n\}$ from the contrast image by using a 3D space-time motion detection algorithm for separating pixels changing values because of motion from those changing values because of contrast flow.

In the second step, the displacements of the selected movement points $p_i \in P$ are computed by means of template matching using the combined invariants-based similarity measure. The new coordinates of the selected control points $p_i \in P$ in the mask image constitute the corresponding set of movement points $Q = \{(x'_i, y'_i),\ i = 1,2,..., n\}$ in this image. Finally, the parameters of the best transformation, which models the deformation between the images, are estimated using the two sets of corresponding movement points (P and Q). The final correction is performed according to this transformation by warping one of the images with respect to the other using the thin- plate spline (TPS) interpolation function [37].

4.1. Movement Points Selection

Determination of the sets P and Q of corresponding movement points is a crucial, and sometimes difficult, task in the registration process. Because the effectiveness of the registration greatly depends on how accurately points are identified, the movement points are automatically extracted by using a 3D space-time motion detection algorithm.

4.1.1. 3D Space-Time Motion Detection Algorithm

Recently, a new, fully automatic motion correction technique was developed, which is capable of aligning pairs of images within few seconds [12]. This technique involves the extraction of the opacified vessels from the background anatomy by an 'a priori' knowledge of the probable variation of arterial iodine concentration with time following an intravenous injection of contrast material.

In this section, we exploit the 3D space-time motion evaluation technique (method 1) for extracting movement points from contrast images. The movement points can be extracted from the contrast images in the sequence by isolating the opacified vessels.

This is done by separating all pixels having their values changed rapidly in time and resulting in only one peak (pixels belonging to opacified vessels) from the unwanted background information (see section 2.2 for a detailed evaluation of this 3-D space-time motion evaluation method).

The first step in the selection of the set P of movement points consists of finding image edges. The location of edges can easily be computed by detecting local maxima of the gray-level gradient magnitude. Since edges are scale dependent image features, they can only be detected properly using derivatives calculated at the proper scale.

The commonly used edge detection filter for this purpose is Gaussian derivative, which allows finer tuning to detect the required edge scale [38].

It should be noted that it is necessary to indicate which edges are important for extracting adequate points. This is done by thresholding the gradient magnitude image at a value S_0, resulting in a binary image in which there are connected regions that are of interest.

Compared to the edge detection approach described in [32], this approach has three major advantages:

1. The number of control points is reduced to an acceptable number of movement points, thereby reducing the required computation time.
2. The application of a 3-D space-time motion detection algorithm enhances the accuracy of movement points extraction and thus the effectiveness of the registration.
3. The movement points are chosen at moving positions where the artifacts can be expected to be the largest.

The following is a summary of the different steps to be followed in the selection of movement points.

1. Compute the gradient magnitude at scale σ of the contrast image. It is based on an edge detection filtering with the application of Gaussian derivative [38].
2. Extract potential artifact regions by means of thresholding the gradient magnitude image at level S_0.
3. Choose a moving window W_m of $w_m \times w_m$ pixels that will sweep over all the pixels in the thresholded edge image. The size of this window depends on the size of the images themselves. This window will be used later for the measure of match.
4. Move the above window, line by line, through the thresholded edge image. If a pixel value is "1" (pixel belonging to an edge), then this pixel is considered to be a control point cp_i.
5. To avoid taking all pixels belonging to an edge inside the same window as control points, take just the central pixel as a control point and, assign a "0" value to all the rest of the pixels in the same window.
6. Repeat steps 4 and 5 until going through all pixels belonging to all edges.
7. For each control point cp_i (pixel belonging to an edge) at position (i, j) in the thresholded edge image, compute vector $\overline{a}_{ij}$:
   - Detect the minimal element of $\overline{a}_{ij}$ according to Equation (3).
   - If this element satisfies conditions (a) and (b) in section 2.2 of method 1 then control point cp_i belongs to a contrasted vessel.
   - Else if this element does not satisfy constraints (a) and (b) in section 2.2 of method 1 then control point cp_i belongs to a moving background anatomy (moving edges), and in this case, it is considered as a movement point p_i.

An example of movement point selection based on this approach is shown in Figure 6.

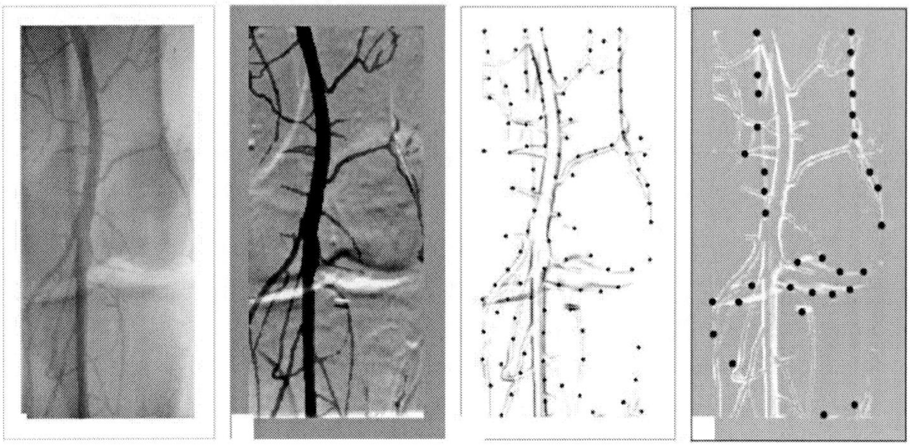

(a) (b) (c) (d)

Figure 6. Movement points selection. (a) A contrast image from a 512 × 512 × 10 digital angiographic image sequence. (b) The subtraction of the contrast image from the mask image showing considerable bone-tissue misregistration. (c) The set of selected control points (black dots), with the edge image superimposed. (d) The set of selected movement points (black dots), with thresholded gradient-magnitude image of the contrast image superimposed. The invalid points (pixels belonging to non moving objects) are removed using the 3-D space-time motion detection algorithm.

4.2. Movement Points Displacements Computation

After extraction of the first set of movement points P in the contrast image, this second step consists of determining the corresponding set of movement points Q in the mask image. For each extracted point $p_i \in P$, a search for its corresponding point $q_i \in Q$ is carried out automatically in a neighborhood beneath it in the other image by template matching. Similarity measures are commonly used to determine the degree of affinity between the two neighborhoods.

The set of combined invariants used in this research are different from the ones used in the second method and are based on image moments and are invariant to symmetric blur, change of contrast, scaling, translation, and rotation. This set is given by the following equations:

$$\Phi_1 = (\nu_{30} - 3\nu_{12})^2 + (3\nu_{21} - \nu_{03})^2 \tag{17}$$

$$\Phi_2 = (\nu_{30} + \nu_{12})^2 + (\nu_{21} + \nu_{03})^2 \tag{18}$$

$$\begin{aligned}\Phi_3 = {} & (\nu_{30} - 3\nu_{12})(\nu_{30} + \nu_{12})\left((\nu_{30} + \nu_{12})^2 - 3(\nu_{21} + \nu_{03})^2\right) + \\ & (3\nu_{21} - \nu_{03})(\nu_{21} + \nu_{03})\left(3(\nu_{30} + \nu_{12})^2 - (\nu_{21} + \nu_{03})^2\right)\end{aligned} \tag{19}$$

$$\Phi_4 = (3\nu_{21} - \nu_{03})(\nu_{30} + \nu_{12})\left((\nu_{30} + \nu_{12})^2 - 3(\nu_{21} + \nu_{03})^2\right) - (\nu_{30} - 3\nu_{12})(\nu_{21} + \nu_{03})\left(3(\nu_{30} + \nu_{12})^2 - (\nu_{21} + \nu_{03})^2\right) \quad (20)$$

$$\Phi_5 = [\nu_{50} - 10\nu_{32} + 5\nu_{14} - 10(\nu_{20}\nu_{30} - \nu_{30}\nu_{02} - 3\nu_{12}\nu_{20} + 3\nu_{12}\nu_{02} - 6\nu_{11}\nu_{21} + 2\nu_{11}\nu_{03})]^2 + [\nu_{05} - 10\nu_{23} + 5\nu_{41} - 10(\nu_{02}\nu_{03} - \nu_{03}\nu_{20} - 3\nu_{21}\nu_{02} + 3\nu_{21}\nu_{20} - 6\nu_{11}\nu_{12} + 2\nu_{11}\nu_{30})]^2 \quad (21)$$

where $\nu_{pq} = \dfrac{\mu_{pq}}{\mu_{00}^{(p+q+2)/2}}$ and $\mu_{pq}^{(I)}$ are the central moments of order $(p+q)$ of the image $I(i,j)$ and $(N \times N)$ is the size of the image.

$$\mu_{pq}^{(I)} = \sum_{i=1}^{N}\sum_{j=1}^{N}\left(i - x_t^{(I)}\right)^p \left(j - y_t^{(I)}\right)^q I(i,j) \quad (22)$$

The coordinates $x_t^{(I)} = \dfrac{m_{10}^{(I)}}{m_{00}^{(I)}}$ and $y_t^{(I)} = \dfrac{m_{01}^{(I)}}{m_{00}^{(I)}}$ denote the centroid of $I(i,j)$.

$m_{pq}^{(I)}$ are the moments of a binary image $I(i,j)$ given by

$$m_{pq}^{(I)} = \sum_{i=1}^{N}\sum_{j=1}^{N} i^p\, j^q\, I(i,j) \quad (23)$$

where $(p+q)$ is the order of moment.

Flusser and Suk [60] showed that these combined invariants are sufficiently robust with respect to noise.

The local displacement of every movement point in the mask image can be estimated over a circular neighborhood of each one of these points detected earlier. After that, the correspondence is established by the minimum distance rule in the Euclidean space of the invariants.

The distance between two circular templates W_1 and W_2 is defined as

$$d_\ell(w_1, w_2) = \left\| \vec{C}(\ell)^{(w_1)} - \vec{C}(\ell)^{(w_2)} \right\| \quad (24)$$

where $\|.\|$ is the Euclidean norm in $l_2(k_\ell)$ space (k_ℓ is the size of $\vec{C}(\ell)$), and the vector $\vec{C}(\ell)$ of combined invariants is defined as

$$\vec{C}(\ell)=(\Phi_1,\Phi_2,...,\Phi_\ell) \tag{25}$$

where ℓ is the number of the combined invariant (here, $\ell = 5$).

In the case of optimal alignment, the distance between the two windows is nil ($d_\ell = 0$).

The displacements of movement points are determined by carrying out the following steps:

1. For every movement point, choose a moving circular template W_1 of radius r centered at this point in the contrast image.
2. Assuming that misregistration parameters would not exceed a 10 pixel shift for image translation (reasonable practical assumptions), calculate the combined invariants vectors $\vec{C}(\ell)^{(W_1)}$ and $\vec{C}(\ell)^{(W_2)}$ of W_1 and the corresponding template W_2 in the mask image, respectively.
3. Calculate the distance d_ℓ between these two templates in the invariant space, taking into consideration the amount of the maximum translational shift. Save the translational shift giving the minimum distance. At the end, the values of the translational shifts will correspond to the displacements of the selected movement points up to integer precision.
4. The movement point $q_i \in Q$ in the mask image that might correspond to the candidate point $p_i \in P$ in the contrast image is determined by the shift position giving the minimum distance.

4.3. Image Warping:

Given the two sets of corresponding movement points, $P = \{p_i\}$ and $Q = \{q_i\}$, the correction is performed by warping the mask image.

In this work mask image warping has been performed by applying the elastic TPS interpolation function [37] on the two sets of movement points as in section 3.3.

4.4. Algorithm 3

The algorithm here is a summary of the operations involved in the registration of two images of a digital angiographic image sequence, presented and discussed in the previous sections.

Given a two-dimensional discrete image sequence $I(x, y, n)$ of size $M \times M \times N$, the registration of a mask image $I(x, y, 0)$ with respect to one of the contrast images $I(x, y, n)$, $n \in [1, N-1] \subset \mathbf{N}$ is accomplished by carrying out the following steps:

1. Using an edge-detection approach based on Gaussian derivative, select the set of control points cp_i in the contrast image $I(x, y, n)$, $n \in [1, N-1] \subset \mathbf{N}$ by following steps 1 to 6 of section 4.1.
2. Using a 3D space-time motion detection algorithm, extract the set of movement points P (points belonging to moving structures) in the contrast image (step 7 of section 4.1).
3. Given the set of movement points P, determine the displacement of every selected movement point $p_i \in P$ using a template matching technique based on the combined invariants-based similarity measure in a circular template of radius r around the selected movement point (steps 1 to 4 of section 4.2).
4. Given the estimated best match position (x_{0i}, y_{0i}) of each movement point p_i, determine the coordinates of the best match, (x_i', y_i'), to subpixel accuracy (Equation (10) of section 3.2.2).
5. Given the two sets P and Q of corresponding movement point pairs in the two images, warp the mask image by using the thin-plate spline (TPS) interpolation function on the two sets of movement points (steps 1 to 3 of section 3.3).

5. Experimental Results

In this section, the performance of the proposed registration technique to the enhancement of DSA images is evaluated experimentally on twenty different X-ray angiography image sequences from five patients (six peripheral, nine cerebral, and five coronary image sequences). The twenty data sets that were used in the experiments consisted of sequences of 512×512 images.

The number of images varies from 10 to 14 for the peripheral and cerebral image sequences and is around 150 for the coronary image sequences. Each image has a gray-value resolution of 8 bits, i.e., 256 gray levels.

The peripheral and cerebral data sets are clinical digital angiographic image sequences, acquired on a DSA imaging system operating at Boston City Hospital, in Massachusetts, and the coronary ones are acquired from a Siemens DSA system operating at Saint Quentin Hospital, in France.

During these experiments, the values of the parameters of the described algorithms were kept fixed to the values specified in [32-34].

5.1. Results of Method 1

The results of applying the proposed detection technique to the two data sets are demonstrated in Figures 7 and 8, respectively. In these figures, six images relate to each data set: (a) the mask image, (b) the contrast image, (c) the original subtraction of the mask image from one of the contrast images, (d) the subtraction after application of a standard pixel-shifting method (registration by global translation of the mask image), (e) the subtraction after correction for patient motion artifacts using the proposed approach and, (f) the subtraction after correction for motion artifacts by applying the proposed approach for all image pixels.

In this implementation the value of the allowable interval of minimal elements (L) around the time of maximum opacification (m) is 2.

From Figures 7 and 8, it can be seen that the artifacts in the image sequences cannot be corrected by applying the pixel shifting technique provided on standard DSA imaging systems (i.e., registration by global translation of the mask image). Clearly, if patient motion is more complex (Figures 7 and 8), a correction in one part of the image implies the introduction of new artifacts in other parts (see Figures 7-d and 8-d).

When comparing these images to the corrected images shown in Figures 7-e and 8-e obtained after applying the proposed approach, it can be clearly seen that most of the motion artifacts have disappeared.

It is obviously noticeable that the application of the proposed correction algorithm when processing all image pixels has given better results than processing only pixels belonging to image edges. In the first case, motion artifacts and gray-level distortions have been removed completely, i.e., the algorithm yields nearly perfect corrections (see Figures 7-f and 8-f). In the second case however, although motion artifacts that appear in those regions of strong object edges have been removed, the correction result still shows some gray-level distortions (see Figures 7-e and 8-e).

It should be mentioned, however, that these small distortions would not reduce the diagnostic value of DSA images. In general with the application of the algorithm to process either image edges (application 1), or the entire image (application 2), most of the misregistration artifacts have disappeared.

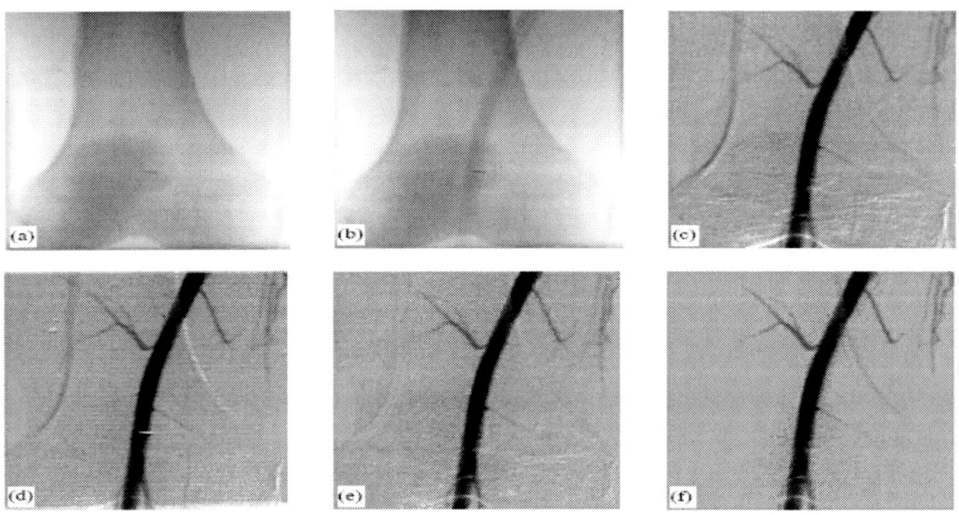

Figure 7. Registration of the first image sequence. (a) Mask image. (b) A contrast image. (c) Original subtraction of the contrast image from the mask image showing considerable bone-tissue misregistration. (d) Registration using the standard pixel-shifting method yielding local correction only (bottom of the image). (e) Registration result using the proposed approach to process only image edges in which most of the artifacts have disappeared. (f) Registration result using the proposed approach to process the entire image yields a perfect subtraction. All the artifacts have disappeared.

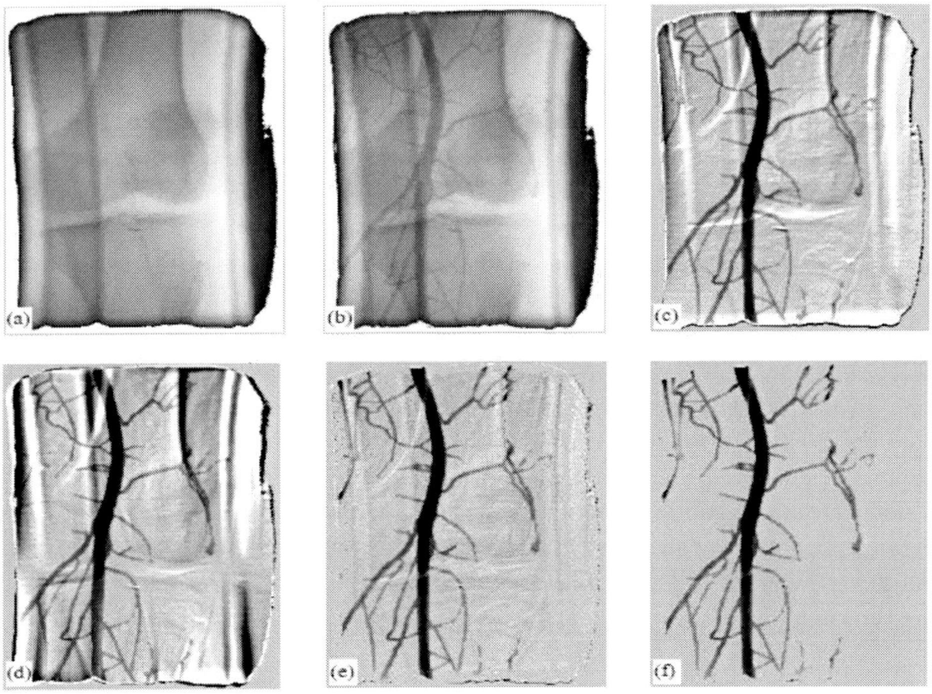

Figure 8. Registration of the second image sequence. (a) Mask image. (b) A contrast image. (c) Original subtraction of the contrast image from the mask image showing considerable bone-tissue misregistration. (d) Registration using the standard pixel-shifting method yielding local correction only (center of the image). (e) Registration result using the proposed approach to process only image edges in which most of the artifacts have disappeared. (f) Registration result using the proposed approach to process the entire image yields a perfect subtraction. All artifacts have disappeared.

When comparing these two applications, the use of the proposed approach to process all image pixels (application 2) generally gives slightly better results than processing only image edges (application 1), while the processing time of that of application 2 takes a little longer than that of application 1. In overall, this proposed approach strongly improves the quality of the subtracted images and correct for motion and gray-level distortion artifacts.

5.2. Results of Methods 2 and 3

In this section, the performance of the second and third registration techniques to the enhancement of DSA image sequences is evaluated experimentally. The results of the application of the proposed registration techniques to a peripheral and a cerebral image sequences are shown in Figures 9 and 10, respectively.

In these figures, seven images are chosen for each data set: (a) the mask image, (b) the contrast image, (c) the registered mask image, (d) the original subtraction of the mask image and the contrast image, (e) the subtraction after application of standard pixel-shifting method (registration by global translation of the mask image), (f) the subtraction after correction for motion artifacts, using method 2, and (g) the subtraction after correction for motion artifacts, using method 3. Figure 9 shows a set of DSA images of a lower extremity (knee) while

Figure 10 shows a set of DSA images of the head. In these sets, bone-tissue artifacts, characterized by sharp whiteness and darkness changes, are very noticeable and really considerable. These artifacts caused by patient motion obscure portions of arteries. It is obvious that such artifacts can lead to misdiagnosis or rejection of the two sets of DSA images. From Figures 9 and 10 it can be seen that the artifacts in the image sequences cannot be corrected by applying the pixel-shifting technique provided on standard DSA imaging systems (i.e., registration by global translation of the mask image). It is clear that if patient motion is more complex, a correction in one part of the image implies the introduction of new artifacts in other parts [11,12].

By comparing these images with the corrected ones after applying the two proposed approaches (method 2 and 3), shown in Figures 9-f, 9-g, 10-f, and 10-g, it can be clearly seen that most of the motion artifacts have disappeared. As can be seen from these images, the proposed algorithms were able to remove the artifacts near the small vessels. Moreover, the application of these two algorithms on a simulated set of coronary artery images (Figure 11) has demonstrated the capability to remove all motion artifacts, even when applied to coronary applications, regardless of the size of the arteries. After this test case, the two registration techniques were applied to a clinical coronary artery sequence. The obtained results for this case are shown in Figure 12.

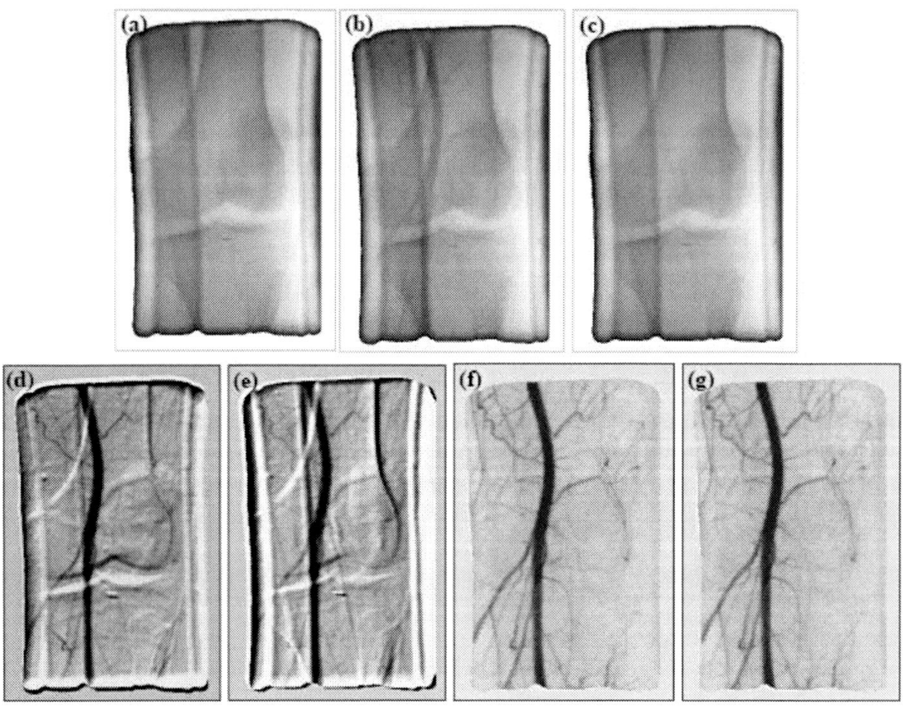

Figure 9. Registration of a peripheral image sequence showing a knee. (a) The mask image. (b) A contrast image. (c) The registered mask image obtained after application of the proposed approach. (d) The original subtraction of the contrast image from the mask image showing considerable bone-tissue misregistration. (e) Registration using standard pixel-shifting method yielding local correction only. (f) The registration result using the second method. Most of the artifacts have disappeared. (g) The registration result using the third approach. Most of the artifacts have disappeared.

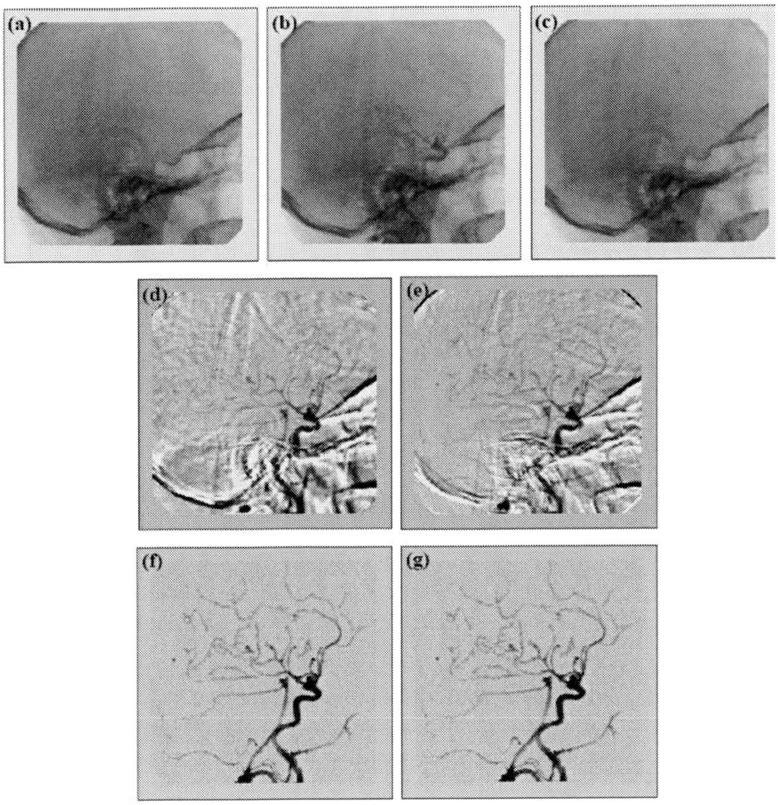

Figure 10. Registration of a cerebral image sequence. (a) The mask image. (b) A contrast image. (c) The registered mask image obtained after application of the proposed approach. (d) The original subtraction of the contrast image from the mask image showing considerable bone-tissue misregistration. (e) Registration using standard pixel-shifting method yielding local correction only. (f) The registration result using the second approach. Most of the artifacts have disappeared. (g) The registration result using the third approach. Most of the artifacts have disappeared.

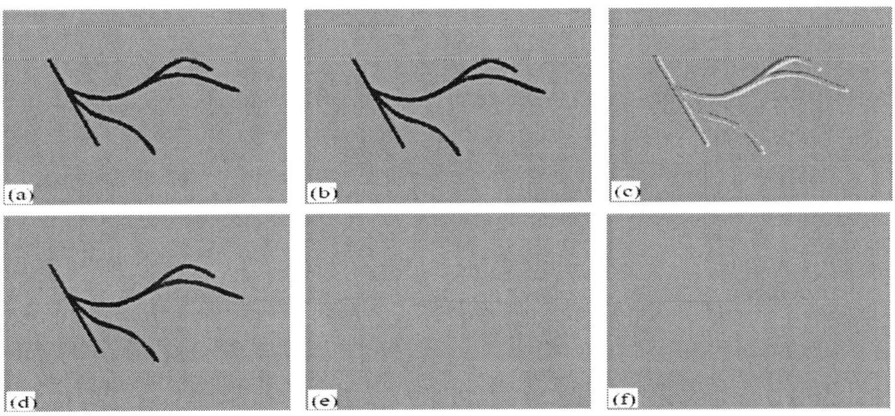

Figure 11. Registration of the simulated set of globally transformed coronary artery images. (a) Image 1. (b) Image 2 (image 1 globally shifted). (c) The difference image between image 1 and image 2. (d) Application of the proposed algorithm to image 2 to register image 1. (e) The difference image after application of the second algorithm. (f) The difference image after application of the third algorithm.

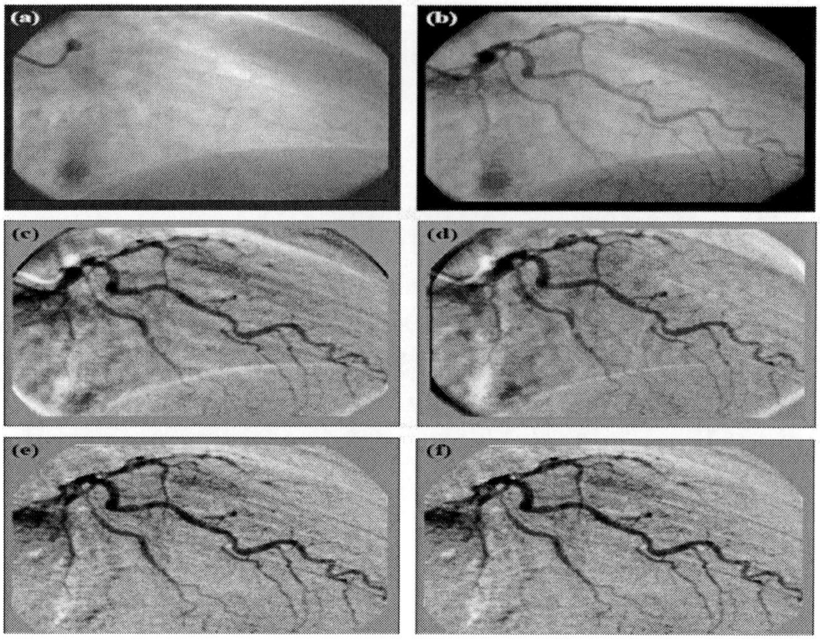

Figure 12. Registration of a coronary image sequence. (a) The mask image. (b) A contrast image. (c) The original difference image showing considerable cardiac motion artifacts. (d) Registration using standard pixel-shifting method yielding local correction only. (e) The registration result using the second approach. Most of the artifacts have disappeared. (f) The registration result using the third approach. Most of the artifacts have disappeared.

From Figure 12-c, it can be seen that motion artifacts, characterized by sharp whiteness and darkness changes in the original subtraction image, are very noticeable and really considerable. These artifacts are due to cardiac contractions and expansions of tissues.

These motion artifacts cannot be corrected by applying the standard pixel-shifting technique (Figure 12-d) because of the complexity of cardiac motion. By comparing these images to the registered one after applying the two automatic methods (Figures 12-e and 12-f), it can be clearly seen that most of the motion artifacts have disappeared. Major vessels are seen to be aligned properly (see Figures 12-e and 12-f).

It is obviously noticeable that there is a small difference between the registration results of peripheral and cerebral image sequences (Figures 9 and 10, respectively) and those of the coronary artery image sequence (Figures 12), when using the proposed method. In the first two sequences, motion artifacts and gray-level distortions have been removed completely, i.e., the algorithm yields nearly perfect registrations. In the coronary image sequence however, although motion artifacts that appear in those regions of strong object edges have been removed, the registration result still shows some gray-level distortions (see Figures 12-e). This is mainly, because the heart cannot be completely modeled as a rigid body. The heart deforms naturally during the cardiac cycle and respiration. It should be mentioned however, that these remaining distortions would not reduce the diagnostic value of the resulting DSA images. In overall, the two invariant registration approaches, based on the combined invariants-based similarity measure and thin-plate spline warping, strongly improve the quality of subtraction images and correct for motion artifacts. An example of extreme cases in which patient motion was large is given in Figure 13.

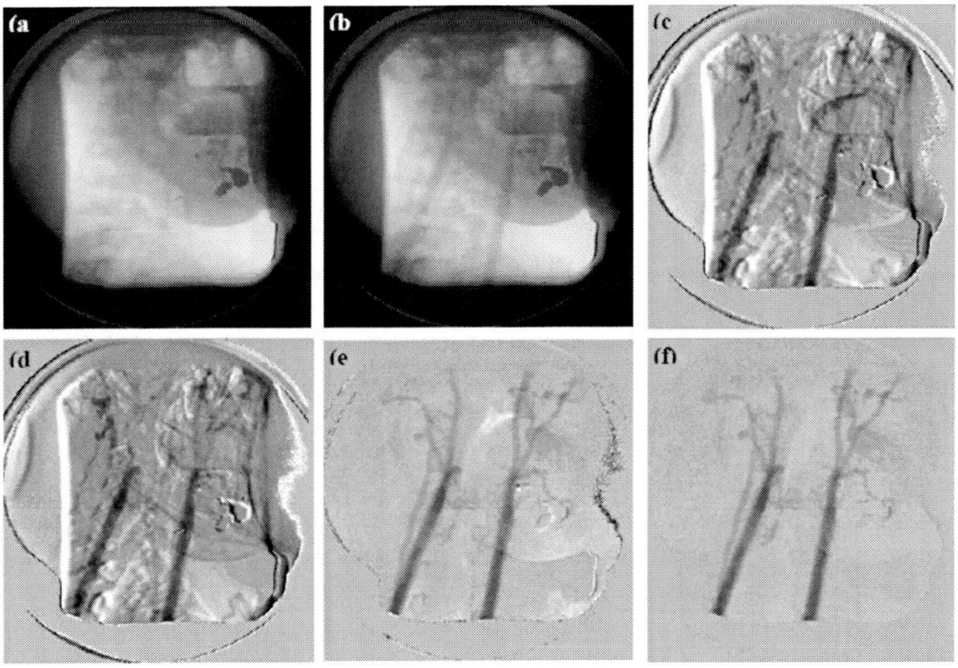

Figure 13. An example of extreme cases in which patient motion was large. (a) The mask image. (b) A contrast image. (c) The original difference image showing considerable patient motion artifacts. (d) Registration using standard pixel-shifting method. Most of the artifacts are still present in the resulting image. (e) The registration result using the second approach. (f) The registration result using the third approach. Most of the artifacts have disappeared.

The difference image shows a substantial amount of motion artifacts around the main vessels, due to considerable movement of the head after the injection of the contrast agent. In this case the manual pixel shifting method was not capable of removing all motion artifacts.

Application of the automatic registration techniques based on the combined invariants resulted in overall correction and improved vessel visibility. The proposed approach, based on the combined invariants-based similarity measure and thin-plate spline warping, strongly improves the quality of subtraction images and provides more useful clinical images than manual pixel shifting. The overall performance of the third registration method was improved by employing a 3-D space-time motion detection for movement point selection in regions where artifacts can be expected to appear and by using thin-plate spline interpolation for image warping. The computational saving with respect to the second method comes from the fact that only pixels belonging to moving edges are processed.

CONCLUSION

This chapter gives a follow-up of three recent automatic registration techniques for digital X-ray angiography images. The main purpose of the first registration technique was to reduce motion artifacts and gray-level distortions by means of blood vessels detection.

The method involves the extraction of a set of control points using an edge-detection approach in an image where artifacts can be expected to appear in the case of patient motion, then, from these control points and by means of the peak iodine opacification detection, this method separates pixels changing values because of motion from those changing values because of contrast flow. This method has led to a new and efficient algorithm that was applied to the worst DSA cases, resulting in images where most of the motion artifacts and gray-level distortions have disappeared.

This algorithm, introducing local processing on areas of interest consisting of pixels belonging to image edges only, is very fast compared to most traditional algorithms.

The second registration method, based on the combined invariants, involves the extraction of a set of control points by using an edge-detection approach to the contrast image where artifacts can be expected to appear in the case of patient motion. The corresponding set of control points in the mask image is determined by means of template matching, using the combined invariants-based similarity measure.

Of all similarity measures developed so far, the combined invariants-based measure was demonstrated to be the most adequate measure for registration of angiographic image sequences. It is insensitive to imperfections of the acquisition system, such as limited spatial resolution, gray-level quantization, blur, noise or the effects of time-varying scatter, and local dissimilarities caused by contrasted vessels. The final correction is accomplished by warping the mask image with respect to each contrast image in the sequence by using thin-plate spline-based interpolation. Moreover, the proposed algorithm demonstrates the capability to remove all motion artifacts when applied to coronary arteries. This algorithm does not assume slowly varying motions only, but also sudden motions. Also the proposed approach yields better global and local registrations, even when applied to the worst DSA cases.

The third registration method is a result of the combination of the two first methods. It involves the extraction of a set of movement points from the contrast image where artifacts can be expected to appear in the case of patient motion. It is based on an edge-detection approach and on a 3-D space-time motion detection algorithm for separating pixels changing values because of motion from those changing values because of contrast flow. The corresponding set of movement points in the mask image is determined by means of template matching, using the combined invariants-based similarity measure.

After establishing the correspondence between small templates in the two images (mask and contrast), the central points of the corresponding templates in the mask image are used as the corresponding set of movement points. The parameters of the affine transformation are computed by using the two sets of corresponding movement points. The final correction is accomplished by warping the mask image with respect to the contrast image by using the thin-plate spline-based interpolation. The proposed registration demonstrates the capability to remove all motion artifacts when applied to coronary arteries. It has been shown to improve the quality of DSA images and to provide more useful clinical images. The algorithm is fully automatic, effective, and computationally efficient when compared to the second algorithm.

The overall results clearly indicate that the third registration algorithm is much better able to recover patient motion than the other ones and would therefore be the method of choice for automatic registration of angiographic images. Moreover, because of the obviously visible high quality of the resulting images, these developed methods may certainly be proposed for implementation and routine use in DSA imaging systems. These efficient algorithms can be used, not only in DSA, but also in any other local or global registration problem as in satellite imaging [61].

REFERENCES

[1] Mistretta, CA; Crummy, AB; Strother, CM. Digital angiography: A perspective. *Radiology,* 1981, vol. 139 No. 2, 273-276.

[2] Brody, WR. Digital subtraction angiography. *IEEE Transactions on Nuclear Science,* March 1982, vol. 29, 1176-1180.

[3] Harrington, DP; Boxt, LM; Murray, PD. Digital subtraction angiography: Overview of technical principles. *Amer. J. Roentgenology*, 1982, vol. 139 No.4, 781-786.

[4] Riederer, SJ; Kruger, RA. Intravenous digital subtraction: A summary of recent developments. Radiology, 1983, vol. 147 No. 3, 633-638: 1983.

[5] Kruger, RA; Riederer, SJ. Basic Concepts of Digital Subtraction Angiography. Boston. MA: G. K. Hall; 1984.

[6] Ovitt, TW; Newell II, JD. Digital subtraction angiography: Technology, equipment, and techniques. *Radiologic Clinics N. Amer.,* 1985, vol. 23 No. 2, 177-184.

[7] Pelz, DM; Fox, AJ; Vinuela, F. Digital subtraction angiography: Curent clinical applications. *Stroke,* 1985, vol. 16 No. 3, 528-536.

[8] Dawson, P. Digital subtraction angiography: A critical analysis. *Clinical Radiology,* 1988, vol. 39 No. 5, 474-477.

[9] Jeans, WD. The development and use of digital subtraction angiography. *Br. J. Radiology,* 1990, vol. 63 No. 747, 161-168.

[10] Katzen, BT. Current status of digital angiography in vascular imaging. *Radiologic Clinics N. Amer.*, 1995, vol. 33 No. 1, 1-14.

[11] Taleb, N; Jetto, L. Image registration for applications in digital subtraction angiography. *Control Engineering Practice,* 1998, vol. 6, 227-238.

[12] Taleb, N; Bentoutou, Y; Deforges, O; Taleb, M. A 3-D space-time motion evaluation for image registration in digital subtraction angiography. *Computerized Medical Imaging and Graphics*, 2001, vol. 25 No. 3, 223-233.

[13] Levin, DC; Shapiro, RM; Boxt, LM; Dunham, L; Harrington, DP; Ergun, DL. Digital subtraction angiography: Principles and pitfalls of image enhancement techniques. *Amer. J. Roentgenology.,* 1984, vol. 143 No. 3, 447-454.

[14] Yanagisawa, M; Shigemitsu, S; Akatsuka, T. Registration of locally distorted images by multiwindow pattern matching and displacement interpolation: The proposal of an algorithm and its application to digital subtraction angiography. In Proc. *Seventh Int. Conf. Pattern Recognition*, 1984, vol. 2, 1288-1291.

[15] Venot, A; Leclerc, V. Automated correction of patient motion and gray values prior to subtraction in digitized angiography. *IEEE Trans. Med. Imag.* April 1984, vol. 3, 179-186.

[16] Takahashi, M; Shinzato, J; Korogi, Y; Fukui, K; Ueno, S; Horiba, I; Suzumura, N. Automatic registration for correction of localized misregistration artifacts in digital subtraction angiography of the head and neck. *Acta Radiologica (Supplementum).*, 1986, vol. 369, 281-284.

[17] Zuiderveld, KJ; Ter Haar Romeny, BM; Viergever, MA. Fast rubber sheet masking for digital subtraction angiography. *In Proc. SPIE,* Bellingham, WA, 1989, vol. 1137, 22-30.

[18] Zuiderveld, KJ; Ter Haar Romeny, BM; Ten Hove, W. Fast techniques for automatic local pixel shift and rubber sheet masking in digital subtraction angiography. In Medical Images: *Formation, Handling and Evaluation*, NATO ASI Series F: Computer and Systems Sciences A.E. Todd-Pokropek, M.A. Viergever, Editors. Berlin, Germany: Springer-Verlag; 1992, vol. 98, 667-685.

[19] Hua, P; Fram, I. Feature-based image registration for digital subtraction angiography. In Proc. SPIE, Bellingham, WA, 1993, vol.1898, 24-31.

[20] Cox, GS; de Jager, G. Automatic registration of temporal image pairs for digital subtraction angiography. *In Proc. SPIE,* Bellingham, WA, 1994, vol. 2167, 188-199.

[21] Buzug, TM; Weese, J; Fassnacht, C; Lorenz, C. Using an entropy similarity measure to enhance the quality of DSA images with an algorithm based on template matching. In Visualization in Biomedical Computing (VBC '96), *Lecture Notes in Computer Science*, K.H. Höhne, R. Kikinis, Editors. Berlin, Germany: Springer-Verlag, 1996, vol. 1131, 235-240.

[22] Buzug, TM; Weese, J. Improving DSA images with an automatic algorithm based on template matching and an entropy measure. In Computer Assisted Radiology (CAR '96), *International Congress Series,* H.U. Lemke, M.W. Vannier, K. Inamura, A.G. Farman, Editors. Amsterdam, The Netherlands: Elsevier; 1996, vol. 1124, 145-150.

[23] Buzug, TM; Weese, J; Lorenz, C; Beil, W. Histogram-based image registration for digital subtraction angiography. In Image Analysis and Processing (ICIAP '97), *Lecture Notes in Computer Science*, A. Del Bimbo, Editor. Berlin, Germany: Springer-Verlag; 1997, vol. 1311, 380-387.

[24] Ko, CC; Mao, CW; Sun, YN. Multiresolution registration of coronary artery image sequences. *Int. J. Med. Informatics*, 1997, vol. 44 No. 2, 93-104.

[25] Buzug, TM; Weese, J. Image registration for DSA quality enhancement. *Computer. Med. Imaging Graphics,* 1998, vol. 22 No. 2, 103-113.

[26] Meijering, EHW; Zuiderveld, KJ; Viergever, MA. A fast technique for motion correction in DSA using a feature-based, irregular grid. In Medical Image Computing and Computer-Assisted Intervention (MICCAI '98), *Lecture Notes in Computer Science,* W. M. Wells, A. Colchester, S. Delp, Editors. Berlin, Germany: Springer-Verlag, 1998, vol. 1496, 590-597.

[27] Meijering, EHW; Zuiderveld, KJ; Viergever, MA. Image registration for digital subtraction angiography. *Int. J. Comput. Vision,* 1999, vol. 31, 227-246.

[28] Digalakis, VV; Ingle, VK; Manolakis, DG. Three-dimensional linear prediction and its application to digital angiography. *Multi-dim. Syst. Sign. Process.,* 1993, vol. 4, 307-329.

[29] Maintz, JBA; Viergever, MA. A survey of medical image registration, *Medical Image Analysis*, 1998, vol. 2, 1-36.

[30] Meijering, EHW; Niessen, WJ; Viergever, MA. Retrospective motion correction in digital subtraction angiography: A review. *IEEE Trans. Med. Imag.,* 1999, vol. 18, 2-21.

[31] Zitova, B; Flusser, J. Image registration methods: A survey, *Image and Vision Computing*, 2003, vol. 21, 977-1000.

[32] Bentoutou, Y; Taleb, N; Chikr El Mezouar, M; Taleb, M; Jetto, L. An invariant approach for image registration in digital subtraction angiography. *Pattern Recognition,* 2002, vol. 35, 2853-2865.

[33] Bentoutou, Y; Taleb, N. Automatic extraction of control points for digital subtraction angiography image enhancement. *IEEE Transactions on Nuclear Science*, February 2005, vol. 52 No. 1, 238-246.

[34] Bentoutou, Y; Taleb, N. A 3-D space-time motion detection for an invariant image registration approach in digital subtraction angiography. *Computer Vision and Image Understanding*, Jan. 2005, vol. 97 No. 1, 30-50.

[35] Rosenfeld, A; Kak, AC. *Digital picture processing. 2nd ed.,* Academic Press, 1982, vol. 1, 245-250.

[36] Simon, JC; Haralick, RM. Digital image processing. *Reidel D. Publishing Company;* 1981, 109-115.

[37] Bookstein, FL. Principal warps: thin-plate splines and the decomposition of deformations. *IEEE-PAMI.,* 1989, vol. 11, 567-585.

[38] Canny, JF. A Computational Approach to Edge Detection. *IEEE Trans. Pattern Analysis and Machine Intelligence*, 1986, vol. 8 No. 6, 679-698.

[39] Barnea, DI; Silverman, HF. A class of algorithms for fast digital image registration. *IEEE Trans. Comput.*, 1972, vol. 21 No. 2, 179-186.

[40] Potel, MJ; Gustafson, DE. Motion correction for digital subtraction angiography. IEEE Frontiers of Engineering and Computing in Health Care: Proceedings of the 5th Annual International Conference of the IEEE Engineering in Medicine and Biology Society; 1983, 166-169.

[41] Pratt, WK. Correlation techniques of image registration. *IEEE Trans. Aerosp. Electron. Syst.*, May 1974, vol. 10, 353-358.

[42] Venot, A; Lebruchec, JF; Roucayrol, JC. A new class of similarity measures for robust image registration. *Comput. Vision Graph. Image Processing,* 1984, vol. 28 No. 2, 176-184.

[43] Venot, A; Golmard, JL; Lebruchec, JF; Pronzato, L; Walter, E; Frij, G; Roucayrol, JC. Digital methods for change detection in medical images. *In Information Processing in Medical Imaging*, F. Deconinck, Ed. Martinus Nijhoff: Dordrecht, The Netherlands; 1984, 1-16.

[44] Van Tran, L; Sklansky, J. Flexible mask subtraction for digital angiography. *IEEE Trans. Med. Imag.*, September, 1992, vol. 11, 407-415.

[45] Wilson, DL; Tarbox, LR; Cist, DB; Faul, DD. Image processing of images from peripheral-artery digital subtraction angiography (DSA) studies. In Proc. SPIE, Bellingham, WA, 1988, vol. 914, 765-771.

[46] Van Tran, L; Sklansky, J. Flexible mask subtraction for digital angiography. *In Proc. SPIE*, Bellingham, WA; 1988, vol. 939, 203-211.

[47] Mandava, VR; Fitzpatrick, JM; Pickens, DR. Adaptive search space scaling in digital image registration. *IEEE Trans. Med. Imag.*, March 1989, vol. 8, 251-262.

[48] Pickens, DR; Fitzpatrick, JM; Grefenstette, JJ; Price, RR; James, AE. A technique for automatic motion correction in DSA. *In Proc. SPIE*, Bellingham, WA, 1986, vol. 626, 268-274.

[49] Fitzpatrick, JM; Pickens, DR; Grefenstette, JJ; Price, RR; James, AE. Techniques for automatic motion correction in digital subtraction angiography. *Opt. Eng.*, 1987, vol. 26 No. 11, 1085-1093.

[50] Fitzpatrick, JM; Pickens, DR; Mandava, VR; Grefenstette, JJ. The reduction of motion artifacts in digital subtraction angiography by geometrical image transformations. *In Proc. SPIE*, Bellingham, WA, 1988, vol. 914, 379-386.

[51] Fitzpatrick, JM; Grefenstette, JJ; Pickens, DR; Mazer, M; Perry, JM. A system for image registration in digital subtraction angiography. In *Image Processing in Medical Imaging*, C. N. de Graaf and M. A. Viergever, Editors. New York: Plenum, 1988, 415-435.

[52] Fitzpatrick, JM; Pickens, DR; Perry, JM; Ge, Y. Experimental results of image registration in digital subtraction angiography with an in vivo phantom. *In Proc. SPIE*, Bellingham, WA, 1989, vol. 1092, 200-213.

[53] Fitzpatrick, JM; Pickens, DR; Chang, H; Ge, Y; Özkan, M. Geometrical transformations of density images. *In Proc. SPIE*, Bellingham, WA, 1989, vol. 1137, 12-21.

[54] Chiang, JY; Sullivan, BJ. Coincident bit counting: A new criterion for image registration. *IEEE Trans. Med. Imag.*, January 1993, vol. 12, 30-38.

[55] Venot, A; Pronzato, L; Walter, E. Comments about the coincident bit counting (CBC) criterion for image registration. *IEEE Trans. Med. Imag.*, March 1994, vol. 13, 565-566.

[56] Lehmann, T; Schmitt, W; Repges, R; Sovakar, A. Mathematical quality standards for digital free-hand subtraction radiography. *Dentomaxillofacial Radiology,* 1995, vol. 24 No. 2, 98.

[57] Buzug, TM; Weese, J; Fassnacht, C; Lorenz, C. Image registration: Convex weighting functions for histogram-based similarity measures. In CVRMed-MRCAS '97, *Lecture Notes in Computer Science,* J. Troccaz, E. Grimson, and R. Mösges, Editors. Berlin, Germany: Springer-Verlag, 1997, vol. 1205, 203-212.

[58] Buzug, TM; Weese, J; Fassnacht, C; Lorenz, C. Elastic matching based on motion fields obtained with a histogram-based similarity measure for {DSA}-image correction. In Computer Assisted Radiology and Surgery (CAR '97), *International Congress Series,* H. U. Lemke, M. W. Vannier, and K. Inamura, Editors. Amsterdam, The Netherlands: Elsevier; 1997, vol. 1134, 139-144.

[59] Buzug, TM; Weese, J; Strasters, KC. Motion detection and motion compensation for digital subtraction angiography image enhancement. *Philips J. Research,* 1998, vol. 51 No. 2, 203-229.

[60] Flusser, J; Suk, T. Degraded image analysis: an invariant approach. *IEEE Trans. Pattern Analysis and Machine Intelligence,* June 1998, vol. 20 No. 6, 590-603.

[61] Bentoutou, Y; Taleb, N; Kpalma, K; Ronsin, J. An automatic image registration for applications in remote sensing. *IEEE Transactions on Geosciences and Remote Sensing*, September 2005, vol. 43 No. 9, 2127-2137.

INDEX

#

A

B

C

D

J

K

L

M

N

O

P

Q

R

S

T